T0227617

MCQs for the New MRCPsych Paper A

with answers explained

Edited by

David Browne, Selena Morgan Pillay,
Guy Molyneaux, Brenda Wright,
Bangaru Raju, Ijaz Hussein,
Mohamed Ali Ahmed and Michael Reilly

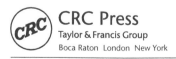

CRC Press
Taylor & Francis Group
Boca Raton London New York

CRC Press is an imprint of the
Taylor & Francis Group, an **informa** business

CRC Press
Taylor & Francis Group
6000 Broken Sound Parkway NW, Suite 300
Boca Raton, FL 33487-2742

International Standard Book Number-13: 978-1-84619-009-4 (Hardback)

Library of Congress Cataloging-in-Publication Data

Names: Browne, David, 1970- , author. | Pillay, Selena Morgan, author.
Title: Master pass MCQs for the new MRCPsych Paper A with answers explained /
David Browne and Selena Morgan Pillay.
Description: Boca Raton : CRC Press/Taylor & Francis, 2016. | Includes
bibliographical references and index.
Identifiers: LCCN 2015042083 | ISBN 9781846190094 (hardback : alk. paper)
Subjects: | MESH: Psychiatry--Examination Questions.
Classification: LCC RC457 | NLM WM 18.2 | DDC 616.890076--dc23
LC record available at http://lccn.loc.gov/2015042083

Visit the Taylor & Francis Web site at
http://www.taylorandfrancis.com

and the CRC Press Web site at
http://www.crcpress.com

CONTENTS

PREFACE v
ABOUT THE EDITORS vii
LIST OF CONTRIBUTORS xi

100 MCQs from Dr. Brenda Wright and Colleagues 1
Dr Olivia Gibbons; Dr Marie Naughton; and Dr Selena Morgan Pillay
References 52

100 MCQs from Dr. Guy Molyneaux and Colleagues 53
Dr Pauline Devitt; Dr Angela Noonan; Dr Klaus Oliver Schubert;
and Prof Finian O'Brien
References 98

100 MCQs from Dr. David Browne and Colleagues 99
Dr Karen Fleming; Dr Michael Kenewali; Dr Manas Sarkar; and Dr Daniel White
References 144

100 MCQs from Dr. Michael Reilly and Colleagues 147
Dr Mohamed Ali Ahmed; Dr Udumaga Ejike; Dr Ijaz Hussein; Dr Atif Ali Magbool;
and Dr Gary McDonald
References 190

INDEX 191

PREFACE

If you are reading this preface, you are unlikely to be casually browsing online or in your local medical bookshop. You are on a mission to complete the MRCPsych examinations. The aim of this book is to help you do just that!

As of Spring 2015, the MRCPsych examination format changed again. Candidates now have to complete two papers rather than three. We have attempted to closely follow the new Paper A curriculum. The book format consists of four best-five questions on one page with the answers explained on the following page to help you clearly understand the subject matter and facilitate learning. All 400 MCQs in this book are referenced with detailed answers, clearly explaining why the answer chosen was the best of the five options available. As the explanatory notes are provided on the next page, there is no need to go hunting through the book looking for the answers. Yes, we have been there! The answers are referenced at the end of each chapter. The references are from the most frequently used examination preparation textbooks and recent or relevant journal articles.

The Royal College of Psychiatrists uses a bank of MCQ questions from multiple authors. In this MCQ book, we have used content from multiple authors, with their varying writing styles, to more accurately reflect the real examination by the Royal College of Psychiatrists. A major advantage of this method is that trainees will gain experience in answering questions that are written in subtly different formats with varying levels of difficulty. There is nothing more demoralising than attempting a set of MCQ questions to discover the questions are uniformly difficult. This is not an accurate reflection of the examination. We believe the format we have chosen along with the detailed explanatory notes will help you acquire the knowledge and skills to be successful at the MCQ component of the Paper A examination.

The authors have donated all royalties from this book to a mental health charity, Shine Supporting People Affected By Mental Ill Health; for more details about the charity, please follow the link, http://www.shineonline.ie.

Finally, the very best of luck with the MRCPsych examination. We wish you every success in your future career in psychiatry!

David Browne and Selena Morgan Pillay,
October 2015

ABOUT THE EDITORS

Dr David Browne, MB, BCH, BAO, DCP, MScLMD, MMEDSc, ACC, MRCPsych
Consultant Psychiatrist, Ashlin Centre, Beaumont Hospital, Dublin 9, Ireland

David Browne qualified in Medicine from University College Galway. He completed the MRCPsych in 2002. He was a Stanley Research Fellow with the Royal College of Surgeons in Ireland and carried out research in the area of epidemiology of first-episode and prevalent psychoses. He has an interest in medical education and training. He was a member of the Royal College of Psychiatrists, Psychiatric Training Committee. He completed a Masters in Medical Education with Queens University Belfast in 2011 and a Masters in Leadership and Management Development with the Royal College of Surgeons in Ireland in 2014. He is a certified coach with the International Coaching Federation. In 2002 he co-authored *MCQs for the New MRCPsych, Part II;* in 2009 he co-authored *MRCPsych Paper 1, One Best Item MCQs*. He is a consultant psychiatrist in Beaumont Hospital, Dublin.

Dr Selena Morgan Pillay, MB, BAO, BCH, DCP, MRCPsych, MMEDSc
Senior Clinical Lecturer RCSI and Consultant Psychiatrist, Beaumont Hospital, Beaumont Rd, Dublin 9, Ireland

Selena Morgan Pillay qualified in Medicine from University College Dublin in 2001. She began basic specialist training in psychiatry with the Dublin University Psychiatric Rotational Training Programme in 2002 and obtained her Membership of the Royal College of Psychiatry in 2005. She completed higher training in General Adult Psychiatry with a special interest in Forensic Psychiatry. During this time, she spent two years working as a Lecturer in Psychiatry, in Trinity College, Dublin, and in the Royal College of Surgeons in Ireland. She obtained a Masters in Medical Education in 2011 from Queens's University Belfast. She is a Senior Clinical Lecturer with the Royal College of Surgeons in Ireland and has been involved in the development of their international psychiatry teaching programmes in Perdana and Bahrain. She is currently working as a Consultant Psychiatrist in Beaumont Hospital.

Dr Guy J. Molyneux, MB, BCH, BAO, MRCPsych, Postgraduate Diploma in CBT, Diploma in Management; Clinical Director in Psychiatry at HSE Dublin North City and County Mental Health Services and MMUH, and Consultant in Adult Psychiatry at St Vincent's Hospital, Fairview, Dublin 3, Ireland

Guy Molyneux received his medical degree (MB BCh BAO) at Dublin University in 1996. He has a special interest in Cognitive Behavioural Therapy and his research on carer burden and mental Illness has been published in national and international scientific journals.

Dr Brenda Wright, MB BCh BAO MRCPsych, MFFLM, Consultant Forensic Psychiatrist
National Forensic Mental Health Service, Dundrum, Dublin 14, Ireland

Brenda Wright qualified in Medicine from UCD in 1997. She completed her psychiatric training with the St John of God Rotation in Dublin, having obtained her Membership of the Royal College of Psychiatry in 2002. She is currently a Consultant in Forensic Psychiatry with the National Forensic Mental Health Service. She previously held the post of Lecturer in Forensic Psychiatry with the National University of Ireland, Trinity College, Dublin. She is a member of the Faculty of Forensic and Legal Medicine of the Royal College of Physicians. She has done research particularly in the areas of psychiatric morbidity in prison and cognitive patterns in sex offenders.

Dr Mohamed Ali Ahmed, MMedSc , MBBS, MRCPsych, DCP, MD
Senior Consultant Psychiatrist and Clinical Director, Adult Community Mental Health Services, Department of Psychiatry, Hamad Medical Corporation, PO Box 3050, Doha, Qatar

Mohamed Ali Ahmed graduated in 1996 and worked in Jordan, Sudan and Saudi Arabia prior to completing his basic psychiatric training on the Western Health Board Psychiatric Training Scheme. He then completed a higher diploma in clinical teaching and participated in teaching postgraduate psychiatric trainees in the west of Ireland. His special interests are transcultural psychiatry, neuroimaging and metabolic disorders in schizophrenia.

Dr Ijaz Hussain, MMedSc, MBBS, MRCPsych, DCP
Consultant Physician, Fraser Health, Surrey Mental Health, Gateway Tower, 11th Floor, Surrey, BC, Canada

Ijaz Hussain graduated in 1999 and worked in Ireland. He completed his basic psychiatric training on the Western Health Board Psychiatric Training Scheme. He developed an interest in teaching as an senior house officer and worked as a Clinical Lecturer with the Department of Psychiatry, National University of Ireland, Galway. He has successfully organised courses for the MRCPsych exam under the old and new curriculum, and is experienced in the recent changes in psychiatric training.

Dr Raju Bangaru, MD, MBA, BS, MRCPsych, DPM
Executive Clinical Director, North Dublin Mental Health Services, Consultant Psychiatrist, Connolly Hospital, Blanchardstown, Dublin 15, Ireland

Raju Bangaru qualified in Medicine from the University of Madras, India, in 1981. He completed basic and higher psychiatric training at the Institute of Psychiatry in Madras. He worked as Assistant Professor of Psychiatry in the University of Madras for nine years. Subsequently, he completed basic and higher psychiatric training in Ireland. His MD (Madras) thesis was on the dexamethasone suppression test. He has completed an MBA in Health Service Management on the UCD/RCSI programme. He has co-authored *MCQs for the New MRCPsych, Part I; MCQs for the New MRCPsych Part II* and *Extended Matching Items for the MRCPsych, Part 1*. His interests include medical education, forensic psychiatry, mood disorders and administration. Since 2006 he has been the Clinical Tutor in Psychiatry of Dublin Northwest Area, and since 2007 he has been the Programme Co-ordinator of RCSI Postgraduate Psychiatric Training Programme. He is the current chair of Continuing Professional Development sub-committee of the Irish College of Psychiatrists.

Dr Michael Reilly, MB, BCh, BAO, MRCPsych, Diploma in Management
Consultant Psychiatrist with a special interest in Rehabilitation Psychiatry, Sligo Mental Health Services, Ballytivnan, Sligo, Ireland

Michael Reilly qualified in Medicine from UCD in 1995. He completed basic specialist training in Psychiatry in 1999 on the Western Health Board Psychiatric Training Scheme. He spent two years researching biological and clinical correlates of suicidal behaviour as part of the INSURE Collaborative Project on suicidal behaviour. He completed higher psychiatric training in the Cavan/Monaghan Mental Health Services and in the Department of Psychiatry, University College Hospital, Galway. He has co-authored a number of MCQ books for the MRCPsych examinations: *MCQs for the New MRCPsych, Part I; MCQs for the New MRCPsych, Part II; Extended Matching Items for the MRCPsych, Part 1* and *MRCPsych Paper 1, One Best Item MCQs*. His interests include medical education, psychiatric ethics and the psycho-social treatment of severe and enduring mental illness.

LIST OF CONTRIBUTORS

Dr Udeme Akpan
*Psychiatrist, Edmonton Mental Health
Services, Alberta Health Service
Edmonton, Alberta, Canada*

Dr Atif Ali Magbool
*Specialist Registrar in Psychiatry, ST5,
The Royal Hospital for Children
Glasgow, Scotland, UK*

Dr Mohamed Ali Ahmed
*Senior Consultant Psychiatrist & Clinical
Director, Adult Community Mental Health
Services, Department of Psychiatry,
Hamad Medical Corporation
Doha, Qatar*

Dr Pauline Devitt
*Consultant Psychiatrist
North Dublin Mental Health Services
Ashlin Centre Beaumont Hospital
Dublin 9, Ireland*

Dr Karen Fleming
*Consultant Old Age Psychiatrist
Cavan/Monaghan Mental Health Services
Monaghan, Ireland*

Dr Olivia Gibbons
*Consultant Psychiatrist
St. Patricks University Hospital
Dublin 8, Ireland*

Dr Ijaz Hussain
*Consultant Physician
Fraser Health, Surrey Mental Health
BC, Canada*

Dr Gary McDonald
*Consultant Child & Adolescent Psychiatrist,
Child and Adolescent Mental Health
Services
Galway, Ireland*

Dr Selena Morgan Pillay
*Senior Clinical Lecturer RCSI & Consultant
Psychiatrist,
Beaumont Hospital, Dublin 9, Ireland*

Dr Marie Naughton
*Consultant Psychiatrist,
St. Patricks University Hospital
Dublin 8, Ireland*

Dr Angela Noonan
*Consultant Psychiatrist
St Vincent's Hospital
Dublin 3, Ireland*

Dr Michael K. Nwali
*Psychiatrist
Medicine Hat Regional Hospital,
Alberta, Canada*

Prof. Finian O'Brien
*Head of Department of Psychiatry
Penang Medical College
Pulau Pinang, Malaysia*

Dr Klaus Oliver Schubert
*Senior Lecturer
Discipline of Psychiatry, School of Medicine,
Lyell McEwin Hospital
University of Adelaide, Adelaide, Australia*

Dr Manas Sarkar
Consultant Child & Adolescent Psychiatrist
Child and Family Consultation Services
Romford, UK

Dr Ejike Udumaga
Consultant Psychiatrist, Mental Health &
Addiction Services
Prince George, Northern Health Authority
BC, Canada

Dr Daniel White
Consultant Psychiatrist with a special
interest in Rehabilitation Psychiatry
North Dublin Mental Health Services
Dublin 9, Ireland

chapter 01

100 MCQs from Dr. Brenda Wright and Colleagues

Dr Olivia Gibbons; Dr Marie Naughton; and Dr Selena Morgan Pillay

1. A 25-year-old woman with a history of schizoaffective disorder has been referred by her GP to your outpatient clinic. She is six weeks pregnant. Her GP requests a review of her medication with regard to teratogenicity. Which of the following medications needs to be most urgently reviewed?

   A. Carbamazepine
   B. Clonazepam
   C. Fluoxetine
   D. Olanzapine
   E. Sodium valproate

2. A 35-year-old man with a diagnosis of schizoaffective disorder is referred by his GP to your outpatient clinic. He is taking risperidone 15 mg daily, having been recently decreased from 20 mg per day. He was noted by his GP to be very restless. He has marked lower limb movement, although he remains seated. He reports sleeping well without a hypnotic. He continues to attend his rehabilitation programme. What is the most likely cause of his restlessness?

   A. Akathisia
   B. Anxiety
   C. Catatonic excitement
   D. Mania
   E. Restless leg syndrome

3. A 33-year-old woman with a history of schizoaffective disorder is referred for assessment by the obstetrics team. She has just given birth to a healthy baby and wishes to breastfeed. They are seeking immediate advice regarding her medication and the risks of breastfeeding. Which of the following medications needs to be most urgently reviewed?

   A. Carbamazepine
   B. Diazepam
   C. Fluoxetine
   D. Olanzapine
   E. Sodium valproate

4. Which of the following factors would help to distinguish the presentation of malingering from factitious disorder?

   A. Lack of cooperation during the diagnostic evaluation.
   B. Lack of cooperation in complying with the prescribed treatment regimen.
   C. Marked discrepancy between the person's claimed stress or disability and the objective findings.
   D. Medicolegal context to presentation.
   E. Presence of antisocial personality disorder.

1. **Answer: E.**

Ideally all medication should be avoided in pregnancy. Polypharmacy should particularly be avoided. Both sodium valproate and carbamazepine are to be avoided in pregnancy, and both have a proven causal link with fetal abnormalities particularly spina bifida. Sodium valproate is regarded as more dangerous than carbamazepine. Benzodiazepines are best avoided in pregnancy, as there is some association with oral clefts in newborns, although there is some debate about the magnitude of this risk. Of the atypical antipsychotics there is most experience with olanzapine, although the risk of gestational diabetes may be increased. Of the SSRIs there is more experience with fluoxetine in pregnancy, although there is an increased risk of premature delivery and reduced birth weight. (1, pp 367–72)

2. **Answer: A.**

Akathisia is distinguished from other causes of restlessness by the prominence of lower limb restlessness. Acute akathisia occurs within hours or weeks of starting antipsychotics or after increasing the dose. It also may occur after a reduction in the dose to treat other extra-pyramidal side effects (EPSE). Risperidone is one of the atypical antipsychotics most strongly associated with EPSEs. Restless leg syndrome is characterised by subjective experience of restlessness interfering with sleep. (1, p 96, 2, p 167, 3, p 487)

3. **Answer: B.**

Repeated doses of long-acting benzodiazepines, such as diazepam, can result in lethargy and weight loss in infants. Carbamazepine is considered low risk in breastfeeding as its levels are relatively low in breast milk. Sodium valproate appears relatively safe, although with a small but finite risk of haematological effects in the infant. Adverse effects have not been reported for most fluoxetine-exposed infants. Olanzapine is excreted in breast milk with infants exposed to about 1% of the maternal dose with no adverse effects. (2, pp 199–206)

4. **Answer: D.**

Malingering differs from factitious disorder in that the motivation for the presentation in malingering is an external incentive, while in factitious disorder external incentives are absent. Factitious disorder would be suggested by evidence of an intrapsychic need to maintain the sick role. (4, pp 309–10)

5. A 20-year-old woman presents to Casualty, having inflicted superficial cuts to her wrists. While waiting to be seen she becomes belligerent and verbally aggressive with staff. She describes recent paranoid ideation and says that she has begun binge eating again in recent months. The current episode of self-harm was precipitated by a row with her boyfriend of three weeks, who she describes as the 'love of my life'. There is a history of unstable employment and relationships. Which is the most likely DSM-IV diagnosis?

    A. Antisocial personality disorder
    B. Borderline personality disorder
    C. Dependent personality disorder
    D. Histrionic personality disorder
    E. Paranoid personality disorder

6. A 22-year-old man is sent for assessment by his GP for depression that is not responding to antidepressant therapy. During the interview, the man reports that from childhood he has wanted to be a girl. He frequently dresses and goes out in public in female clothing. He reports that he is sexually attracted to men, which he believes is evidence of the wrong gender assignment. He has no paraphilic interests. What is the most likely diagnosis?

    A. Egodystonic sexual orientation
    B. Fetishism
    C. Gender identity disorder
    D. Polymorphously perversion
    E. Transvestic fetishism

7. A 65-year-old single man presents with a history of alcohol dependence syndrome. He recently relapsed, drinking approximately 20 units of alcohol per day for the past two months. He has not had a drink in 24 hours. He has a history of seizures on one previous occasion when withdrawing from alcohol. Which of the following is the most appropriate approach to his management?

    A. Inpatient detoxification with chlordiazepoxide, carbamazepine and parenteral thiamine.
    B. Inpatient detoxification with chlordiazepoxide and parenteral thiamine.
    C. Outpatient detoxification with chlordiazepoxide.
    D. Outpatient detoxification with chlordiazepoxide and carbamazepine.
    E. Outpatient detoxification with chlordiazepoxide, carbamazepine and oral thiamine.

8. A 19-year-old man presents to Casualty seeking detoxification from benzodiazepines. He reports that he has been taking diazepam 50 mg daily. He says that he has not taken any in 48 hours and says that he is experiencing withdrawal symptoms. Which of the following symptoms is he most likely to describe?

    A. Anxiety symptoms
    B. Decreased consciousness
    C. Extreme fatigue
    D. Runny nose and eyes
    E. Vomiting

5.   Answer: B.

This woman demonstrates the following features of borderline personality disorder:

A pattern of unstable and intense interpersonal relationships. Recurrent suicidal behaviour, gestures or threats as well as self-mutilating behaviour. Transient stress-related paranoid ideation. Impulsivity as characterised by her binge eating and substance abuse. Inappropriate, intense anger or difficulty controlling anger. She may demonstrate traits of other Cluster B personality disorders such as antisocial personality disorder: impulsivity or failure to plan ahead, irritability and aggressiveness.

Histrionic personality disorder: considers relationships to be more intimate than they actually are, shows self-dramatisation and exaggerated expression of emotion. (4, pp 291–3)

6.   Answer: C.

Gender identity disorder is characterised by a strong and persistent cross-gender identification marked by the stated desire to be the other sex, frequent passing as the other sex and a desire to live or be treated as the other sex. In egodystonic sexual orientation the patient states that the sustained pattern of homosexual arousal is unwanted and is a source of distress. There is a desire to acquire heterosexual orientation. Fetishism involves sexual arousal to non-living objects and is a type of paraphilia. Polymorphous perversion is the harbouring of more than one form of paraphilia. (4, pp 259–61, 5, pp 251–3)

7.   Answer: E.

Elderly patients with a history of withdrawal seizures should be detoxified as inpatients. All inpatient detoxification regimes should include prophylactic parenteral thiamine for Wernicke's encephalopathy as there is limited evidence for oral thiamine. There is no definitive evidence for the use of anticonvulsants for alcohol withdrawal. (1, pp 304, 313–14)

8.   Answer: A.

Extreme fatigue is more characteristic of withdrawal from amphetamines. Decreased consciousness is more characteristic of withdrawal from cocaine. Runny nose and eyes (rhinitis) is more characteristic of withdrawal from heroin. Vomiting is more characteristic of withdrawal from alcohol or barbiturates. (1, p 346)

9. A 46-year-old married man with a history of dysthymia presents in the outpatient department complaining of impotence. Which of the following medications is the most likely cause of this problem?

   A. Clomipramine
   B. Mirtazapine
   C. Phenelzine
   D. Reboxetine
   E. Venlafaxine

10. A 25-year-old woman with a diagnosis of depression is reviewed in the outpatient department. She anxiously describes the experience of hearing voices at night in bed while she goes to sleep. Which of the following perceptual abnormalities is this woman most likely experiencing?

   A. Extracampine hallucinations
   B. Hypnagogic hallucinations
   C. Hypnopompic hallucinations
   D. Pseudohallucinations
   E. Reflex hallucinations

11. A 45-year-old woman presents for assessment, describing a long history of anxiety when out in public. She recalls the onset of her difficulties when, as a 20-year old, she experienced her first panic attack. She avoids social events and in recent times is leaving her home much less frequently. She says that she is fearful of experiencing a panic attack away from home, although she has not had a panic attack in over three months. Which is the most likely diagnosis in this case according to DSM-IV criteria?

   A. Agoraphobia with a history of panic disorder
   B. Generalised anxiety disorder
   C. Panic disorder with agoraphobia
   D. Separation anxiety disorder
   E. Social phobia

12. Which of the following syndromes is least associated with a psychotic illness?

   A. Couvade syndrome
   B. De Clerambault's syndrome
   C. Fregoli's syndrome
   D. Othello syndrome
   E. Syndrome of subjective doubles

9. **Answer: E.**

The approximate prevalences of sexual side effects with antidepressants are as follows:

Tricyclic antidepressants	30%
Reboxetine	5–10%
Mirtazapine	25%
MAOIs	40%
Venlafaxine	70%

10. **Answer: B.**

Hypnagogic hallucinations occur while going asleep. Hypnopompic hallucinations occur on waking. Sims (1998) comments that the importance of these phenomena is in recognising their existence and realising that they are not necessarily abnormal although they may be truly hallucinatory. Reflex hallucinations occur when a stimulus in one modality produces a hallucination in another. A pseudohallucination is a perceptual experience that is figurative, not concretely real, and occurs in inner subjective space, not in external objective space. Extracampine hallucinations are experienced by the patient as outside the limits of the sensory field. (5, p 96)

11. **Answer: C.**

DSM-IV classifies the following disorders: panic disorder without agoraphobia, panic disorder with agoraphobia, agoraphobia without a history of panic disorder. Agoraphobia is not a codable disorder, so there is no diagnosis of agoraphobia with panic disorder. Therefore this woman has panic disorder with agoraphobia. Her avoidance of public situations is provoked by the fear of a panic attack rather than a fear of social performance which would characterise a social phobia. In generalised anxiety disorder there is excessive anxiety and worry occurring more days than not for at least six months. The focus of the anxiety is not confined to features of an Axis I disorder, e.g. the anxiety or worry is not about having a panic attack. Separation anxiety disorder has an onset before the age of 18 years. (4, pp 77, 209–16)

12. **Answer: A.**

In Couvade syndrome a person develops extreme anxiety and various physical symptoms of pregnancy when their partner is pregnant. The partner may have morning sickness, abdominal pains, constipation, food craving and so on. It is thought to be a manifestation of anxiety. It may be an expression of frustrated creativity, jealousy of the attention paid to the pregnant partner or over-identification with the pregnant partner. It is usually managed with reassurance. In Fregoli's syndrome the patient believes that ordinary people in his environment are persecutors in disguise. In De Clerambault's syndrome the patient believes that another person loves him intensely. The object of the delusion is often of higher social status. Othello syndrome involves delusion of infidelity on the part of a sexual partner. In the syndrome of subjective doubles the patient believes that doubles of himself exist. (6, pp 160–3)

13. A 65-year-old right-handed man is seen in hospital following a cerebrovascular accident. At interview he is noted to have significant difficulties with comprehension. He is also noted to speak fluently but with numerous errors in the use of words, syntax and grammar. Which of the following best describes the location of the cortical lesion in this man's case?

A. Right frontal lobe
B. Left angular gyrus
C. Left premotor cortex
D. Left temporal lobe
E. Right temporal lobe

14. A 35-year-old man with schizoaffective disorder presents with urinary retention. Which of the following medications is most likely to be responsible?

A. Carbamazepine
B. Clomipramine
C. Clonazepam
D. Haloperidol decanoate
E. Lithium

15. An advertising company is planning a campaign for an alcoholic beverage. The television advertisement shows a tropical beach. Two actors then walk along the sand drinking the alcoholic beverage. What type of conditioning is the advertising company using in this advertising campaign?

A. Backward conditioning
B. Higher order conditioning
C. Simultaneous conditioning
D. Stimulus generalisation
E. Trace conditioning

16. A researcher wishes to evaluate the attitudes of the general public to people with mental health problems. He designs a questionnaire using a Likert scale. What is the most likely source of bias associated with the use of this questionnaire?

A. Bias to middle
B. Defensiveness
C. Halo effect
D. Hawthorn effect
E. Response set

17. A 65-year-old man is referred for assessment by the cardiology team. He has a history of unstable angina and has become depressed. Which of the following antidepressants would be the most suitable for treating this man's depressive episode?

A. Clomipramine
B. Mirtazapine
C. Phenelzine
D. Reboxetine
E. Venlafaxine

13. **Answer: B.**

This man has Wernicke's dysphasia (sensory or receptive dysphasia), resulting from a lesion to the angular gyrus in the posterior part of the superior gyrus of the dominant temporal lobe. Broca's dysphasia (expressive or motor dysphasia) results from a lesion to the precentral gyrus in the dominant frontal cortex. In 90% of right-handed people the left hemisphere plays the predominant role in speech. Wernicke's dysphasia can be distinguished from Broca's dysphasia by the fluency of speech. (5, pp 159–63)

14. **Answer: B.**

Urinary retention is an anticholinergic side effect. Clomipramine is one of the most potent anticholinergic medications. Lithium is more likely to cause polyuria. Haloperidol decanoate can cause anticholinergic side effects but has less potential than clomipramine. Benzodiazepines are not uncommonly used postoperatively to reduce urinary retention. There are isolated case reports of urinary retention with carbamazepine but this is not a common side effect. (2, pp 162, 166, 217)

15. **Answer: A.**

Backward conditioning involves the introduction of the conditioned stimulus (CS, the drink) after the unconditioned stimulus (UCS, the tropical beach). Trace conditioning: the CS is presented and removed before the UCS so only a memory of the CS remains. Simultaneous conditioning: the CS and the UCS are presented together. Stimulus generalisation: two similar CS can generate the same conditioned response (CR). Higher order conditioning: the CS can be paired with another stimulus to produce a further CR. The original CS serves as a UCS for the new association. (7, p 74)

16. **Answer: A.**

Responders on Likert scales are more likely to show a bias to the middle or the avoidance of extreme responses. Responders to a questionnaire on mental illness might also demonstrate the halo effect, allowing preconceptions to influence their responses. However this is not the result of the Likert scale design of the questionnaire. (7, p 92)

17. **Answer: B.**

Tricyclics and venlafaxine are the highest risk in treating patients with cardiac disease. MAOIs and reboxetine pose a moderate risk. Mirtazapine along with the SSRIs is believed to pose the lowest risk in patients with cardiac problems. (2, p 207)

18. A 44-year-old man is attending for treatment of bipolar affective disorder. A routine blood investigation reveals a raised ALP and gamma GT. Which of the following drugs is most likely to have caused this abnormality?

A. Carbamazepine
B. Haloperidol
C. Lithium
D. Olanzapine
E. Sodium valproate

19. A 50-year-old woman is attending for treatment of bipolar affective disorder. She has been on lithium for ten years. Which of the following blood profiles is most likely in this woman?

A. Ca^{2+} ↑ Phosphate ↓
B. Ca^{2+} ↓ Phosphate ↑
C. T4 ↓ T3 ↑ TSH ↓
D. T4 ↑ T3 ↓ TSH ↓
E. T4 ↑ T3 ↑ TSH ↑

20. A 30-year-old man with diabetes mellitus is referred by his general practitioner for treatment of a depressive episode. Which of the following antidepressants would be the most suitable?

A. Clomipramine
B. Fluoxetine
C. Mirtazapine
D. Phenelzine
E. Sertraline

21. A 22-year-old woman is referred by her general practitioner who reports that she has anorexia nervosa. Following your assessment, you are of the opinion that this woman has bulimia nervosa. Which of the following features in her history would most support your diagnosis?

A. Binging episodes
B. Body mass index 22.5
C. Morbid fear of fatness
D. Persistent preoccupation with eating
E. Self-induced vomiting

22. A 35-year-old married man, who is long-term unemployed, is referred for psychiatric assessment. He is accompanied by his wife. He was attacked three months ago by two men who drove him around in the boot of a car for two hours before holding a gun to his head and threatening to shoot him. He was then beaten and left on the side of the road. You diagnose a post-traumatic stress disorder. He also has a history of depressive disorder. Which of the following features in this man's case would most likely improve his prognosis?

A. Duration of the trauma
B. Premorbid function
C. Psychiatric history
D. Severity of the trauma
E. Social support

18. **Answer: A.** A raised ALP and gamma GT are potentially a sign of a hypersensitivity reaction to carbamazepine. Sodium valproate may very rarely cause fulminant hepatic failure, although all cases to date have occurred in children, often receiving multiple anticonvulsants with family histories of hepatic problems. (1, p 154)

19. **Answer: A.** A raised Ca^{2+} and a lowered phosphate are characteristics of hyperparathyroidism that can be caused by long-term lithium therapy. Hypothyroidism, also caused by long-term lithium therapy, would be characterised by a raised T4, a raised T3 and a lowered TSH. None of these thyroid profiles is represented in the options. (2, pp 379–82)

20. **Answer: E.** The antidepressant of choice in a patient with diabetes is sertraline. Fluoxetine can cause hypoglycaemia, and its side effects (tremor, sweating, nausea, anxiety) may be mistaken for hypoglycaemia. MAOIs may reduce serum glucose by up to 30% by their direct influence on the pathway of gluconeogenesis. Tricyclics may adversely affect diabetic control as they increase serum glucose levels by up to 150%, increase carbohydrate craving and reduce the metabolic rate. The manufacturers of mirtazapine recommend care, although there are no reports of problems. (2, pp 215–7)

21. **Answer: B.** Bulimia nervosa and anorexia nervosa share a number of features, including a morbid fear of fatness, a preoccupation with eating, vomiting or purging behaviour and binge eating. The diagnosis of anorexia requires a BMI of <17.5, and amenorrhea. It should be remembered, however, that 15% of patients with anorexia progress to bulimia. (6, pp 93–100)

22. **Answer: E.** Good prognostic factors in post-traumatic stress disorder are a healthy premorbid function, a brief trauma of lesser severity, no personal history of psychiatric illness and good social support. In this man's case, he has a number of poor prognostic factors; however, he appears to have the support of his partner. (6, p 74)

23. You have been seeing a 45-year-old man who presented with symptoms of depressive disorder and post-traumatic symptoms following an accident at work. He has shown little response to antidepressant medication at high doses, and the diagnosis remains unclear. You refer him for psychological assessment. Which of the following instruments would you most likely expect the psychologist to use?

A. Adaptive Behaviour Scales
B. Brief Psychiatric Rating Scale
C. CAGE Questionnaire
D. General Health Questionnaire
E. Minnesota Multiphasic Personality Inventory

24. A 22-year-old patient presents with a movement disorder. He demonstrates rapid sudden blinking. This movement is more noticeable when the patient is anxious. His partner reports that it does not occur when he is asleep, and that it is less prominent when he is concentrating on an activity. Which movement is this patient most likely displaying?

A. Dyskinesia
B. Hemiballismic movements
C. Myoclonic movements
D. Tics
E. Torticollis

25. A 35-year-old married woman with a history of depressive disorder presents in the outpatient department complaining of loss of libido. Which antidepressant medication would be the most suitable to prescribe to address this side effect?

A. Fluoxetine
B. Lofepramine
C. Phenelzine
D. Mirtazapine
E. Venlafaxine

26. A 24-year-old woman with a diagnosis of schizophrenia presents to the outpatient department. She reports that she is being sexually assaulted every night by terrorists. Which of the following perceptual abnormalities is she most likely to be experiencing?

A. Autoscopic hallucinations
B. Haptic hallucinations
C. Hygric hallucinations
D. Hypnagogic hallucinations
E. Kinaesthetic hallucinations

23. **Answer: E.**

The Minnestoa Multiphasic Personality Inventory (MMPI) is a self-rated questionnaire validated on psychiatric patients not normal given 'personality profile'. The Adaptive Behaviour Scales are used in patients with intellectual disability. The Brief Psychiatric Rating Scale is used to measure psychotic symptoms and psychopathology. The CAGE is a brief screening tool for alcohol abuse. The General Health Questionnaire is a commonly used screening tool used in primary care and general population studies. (6, pp 6–8)

24. **Answer: D.**

Tics are rapid, purposeless movements of a functionally related group of muscles. They are most commonly facial. They increase with anxiety and decrease during sleep. They may be reduced during periods of sustained attention. Myoclonic movements may be distinguished from tics as they affect a whole muscle or part of a muscle but not muscle groups. Dystonic movements are slower and more sustained than tics. Hemiballismic movements are movements of the limbs, which are coarse, intermittent and unilateral. Dyskinetic movements that tend to occur in the facial muscles, e.g., tardive dyskinesia, also affect muscle groups but are slower than tics. Torticollis involves the gradual development of tonic spasms in the neck muscles. (6, p 285)

25. **Answer: D.**

Mirtazapine has a lower incidence of sexual side effects than most other antidepressants at 24%. SSRIs may indirectly decrease libido through a direct inhibition of sexual arousal and orgasm. Tricyclic antidepressants may decrease libido indirectly through sedation. Venlafaxine can inhibit arousal and orgasm. (2, pp 195–7)

26. **Answer: B.**

Haptic hallucinations are superficial hallucinations of touch. The hallucination may be delusionally elaborated. Hygric hallucinations are superficial hallucinations of fluid. Kinaesthetic hallucinations are those of muscle or joint sense. Hypnagogic hallucinations are perceptions that occur while going asleep. Autoscopic hallucinations are abnormalities of visual perceptions involving seeing oneself. (5, pp 89–90)

27. A 26-year-old man is seen following a road traffic accident in which he sustained serious head and limb injuries. He is noted to have a palsy in his left arm. Which of the following features would most likely suggest that the upper-limb paralysis results from an upper rather than a lower motor neuron lesion?

A. Babinski sign
B. Fasciculation
C. Flaccid paralysis
D. Hyporeflexia
E. Hypotonia

28. A 56-year-old man with a history of alcohol dependence syndrome is referred by the Accident and Emergency Registrar who reports that he has Wernicke's encephalopathy. Following your assessment, you are of the opinion that he has progressed to Korsakoff's syndrome. Which of the following features would be most supportive of your diagnosis?

A. Confabulation
B. Confusion/Clouding of consciousness
C. Nystagmus
D. Peripheral neuropathy
E. Staggering gait

29. A 36-year-old woman attends for assessment at the outpatient clinic. She reports that she has been previously diagnosed with 'seasonal affective disorder'. Which of the following features of her depressive disorder is least supportive of this diagnostic term?

A. Hyperphagia
B. Insomnia
C. Loss of interest
D. Low energy
E. Symptoms worsening in the months of November to February

30. A 25-year-old man who has been attending the service for treatment of anxiety disorder is involved in a road traffic accident. Which of the following factors increases this man's risk for significant cognitive sequelae?

A. Glasgow Coma Scale (GCS) score of 13 following the accident
B. No intracranial bleeding
C. Non-penetrating injury
D. Post-traumatic amnesia of 5–6 days
E. Retrograde amnesia covering minutes before the accident

27. **Answer: A.** An upper motor neuron lesion will be characterised by hypertonia, spastic paralysis, hyperreflexia and the Babinski sign. A lower motor neuron lesion will be characterised by hypotonia, flaccid paralysis, hyporeflexia and muscles wasting with fasciculation and fibrillation. (7, p 29)

28. **Answer: A.** Korsakoff's syndrome is characterised by the inability to form new memories and retrograde amnesia, confabulation, relative preservation of other intellectual functions, clear consciousness and peripheral neuropathy. The presentation of Wernicke's encephalopathy also involves peripheral neuropathy, with ocular palsies and nystagmus, ataxia, confusion and clouding of consciousness. (6, p 125)

29. **Answer: B.** Seasonal affective disorder was a term used to describe patients who recognised a seasonal pattern to their mood and described consistent atypical symptoms of hypersomnia, hyperphagia, tiredness and low mood in winter. Community studies have not supported the existence of a specific syndrome, although there is some seasonality in mood disorder. (8, p 407)

30. **Answer: E.** A post-traumatic amnesia of 1–7 days indicates severe injury. A Glasgow Coma Score of 13–15 suggests mild injury. The shorter the period of retrograde amnesia, the less severe the injury. A penetrating head injury and intracranial bleeding would worsen the prognosis, but this man sustained neither. (6, p 193, 8, pp 309–10)

31. A 36-year-old man who is being treated for depressive disorder complains that he has been experiencing sleep difficulties. He reports that his wife complains he appears frightened and shouts in his sleep at night. He has no recollection of the incidents on waking. Which type of sleep disturbance is this man most likely describing?

   A. Narcolepsy
   B. Night terrors
   C. Nightmares
   D. Sleep drunkenness
   E. Somnambulism

32. Which of the following symptoms is least likely characteristic of temporal lobe epilepsy?

   A. Automatism
   B. Déjà vu
   C. Echolalia
   D. Olfactory hallucinations
   E. Pseudohallucinations

33. A male patient with Tourette's syndrome is referred to the clinic for assessment. The referring doctor reports that in addition to vocal tics, he has a number of other psychiatric difficulties associated with Tourette's. Which of the following symptoms is this patient least likely to display?

   A. Anxiety
   B. Attention deficits
   C. Depressive episode
   D. Obsessional symptoms
   E. Psychotic symptoms

34. A 55-year-old man presents with sudden onset unilateral facial paralysis. The upper and lower facial muscles are equally affected. The eyebrow droops and the wrinkles of the forehead are smoothed out. The muscles are equally affected for voluntary, emotional and associated movements. There is loss of taste on the anterior two-thirds of the tongue. The patient is well otherwise. Which of the following is the most likely diagnosis in this case?

   A. Bell's palsy
   B. Horner's syndrome
   C. Multiple sclerosis
   D. Poliomyelitis
   E. Ramsay–Hunt syndrome

31. **Answer: B.**

Night terrors occur in deep sleep early in the night. They more typically occur in childhood, but can occur in adulthood. The person displays intense anxiety, may shout, and has a rapid pulse and respiration. Usually there is complete amnesia for the experience on waking. This latter point distinguishes night terrors from nightmares, a type of dream that is remembered vividly if the person awakes immediately after the experience. Narcolepsy is characterised by short episodes of sleep that occur irresistibly during the day. Somnambulism is another term for sleepwalking. Sleep drunkenness is the complaint of feeling drowsy, incompetent and uncoordinated for a prolonged period of time on waking. (5, pp 40–3)

32. **Answer: C.**

Echolalia, the repetition of words or parts of sentences that are spoken in the patient's presence, more typically occurs in schizophrenic states, intellectual disability and dementia. It is not part of the profile of temporal lobe epilepsy. An automatism is an action taking place in the absence of consciousness and is characteristic of temporal lobe epilepsy. Pseudohallucinations may occur as autoscopy in temporal lobe epilepsy. Déjà vu and olfactory hallucinations can occur as part of the aura in temporal lobe epilepsy. Visual hallucinations may occur as part of the seizure. (5, pp 32, 88, 92, 95)

33. **Answer: E.**

Patients with Tourette's syndrome have been found to have an increased prevalence of depressive, anxiety and obsessional symptoms than normal controls. There is additionally an increased prevalence of deliberate self-harm. There does not appear to be any association with increased psychotic symptoms. (5, p 341, 6, p 287)

34. **Answer: A.**

Bell's palsy is diagnosed by the sudden onset of a unilateral facial paralysis with or without loss of taste in the anterior two-thirds of the tongue in a person who is otherwise well. Ramsay–Hunt syndrome occurs with herpes zoster of the geniculate ganglia. There is a facial palsy identical to Bell's palsy but with herpetic lesions in the external auditory meatus. Deafness may occur. Multiple sclerosis should be considered as a possible cause when unilateral facial paralysis occurs in a young adult, especially if it is painless, not very severe and clears up in two or three weeks. Poliomyelitis should be considered as a cause when unilateral facial paralysis occurs during an epidemic of that disease, especially in a child or adolescent, and if it occurs a few days after a febrile illness. (3, p 888, 9, pp 67–9)

35. A 36-year-old woman who was diagnosed with puerperal psychosis attends the outpatient department accompanied by her husband. They would like to have more children but want to know what the chances are of the illness recurring. Which of the following figures best represents this woman's chance of becoming psychotic again following childbirth?

A. 1%
B. 5%
C. 10%
D. 20%
E. 30%

36. A 22-year-old woman has been referred to the neurology service for assessment. She was initially referred to a neurologist for treatment of seizures; however, the neurologist is of the opinion that she is not experiencing true seizures. Which of the following features most likely suggests that this woman is presenting with non-epileptic seizures?

A. Extensor plantar reflexes following the seizure
B. Incontinence
C. Increased seizure activity when attempts made to restrain the patient
D. Loss of corneal reflexes during and following the seizure
E. Tonic-clonic seizures

37. A patient reports that he has been experiencing visual hallucinations. He describes seeing the face of his sister in the clouds. Which of the following perceptual abnormalities is this man most likely experiencing?

A. Affect illusion
B. Completion illusion
C. Elementary hallucination
D. Functional hallucination
E. Pareidolic illusion

38. A 22-year-old woman is referred for assessment by the obstetric team. She is reported to be feeling depressed following the birth of her first baby three days ago. She has no history of depressive disorder. The baby is healthy, although the woman required a caesarean delivery. Which of the following is the most likely diagnosis?

A. 'Baby blues'
B. Adjustment disorder
C. Adjustment reaction
D. Major depressive episode with post-partum onset
E. Major depressive disorder

35.   **Answer: E.**   Women who experience a puerperal psychosis have a one in three chance of a further psychotic episode following a subsequent pregnancy. This woman's risk would be further increased by a personal or family history of a major mental disorder. Risk is higher in women with a history of bipolar rather than unipolar affective disorder. (8, p 560)

36.   **Answer: C.**   Non-epileptic seizures occur very commonly in patients who also experience epileptic seizures. The movements in non-epileptic seizures often involve generalised rigidity with arching of the back and random thrashing of the limbs, contrasting with the stereotypical tonic-clonic movements in grand mal seizures. Reflexes are unaltered in non-epileptic attacks. Incontinence is common in epileptic seizures but rare in non-epileptic episodes. (8, p 31)

37.   **Answer: E.**   There are three type of illusions. A completion illusion occurs when an incomplete perception that is meaningless in itself is filled in a process of extrapolation from a previous experience to produce significance. An affect illusion is one that can be understood in the context of the person's mood state, for example when a child frightened by the dark mistakes a blowing curtain for a person in the room. Pareidolic illusions are created out of sensory percepts by an admixture with imagination. Functional hallucinations occur when a certain percept is necessary for the production of a hallucination but the hallucination is not a transformation of that percept. For example, the patient hears voices when a tap is turned on. An elementary hallucination is an auditory hallucination of unstructured sounds, often occurring in an organic state. (5, pp 81–5)

38.   **Answer: A.**   Baby blues typically occur 3–6 days following the birth of the baby in 50–60% of mothers. Post-partum depression occurs in approximately 10% of women after parturition. It usually occurs within 6–8 weeks of birth, most often beginning between days 3 and 14 after parturition. Adjustment disorder is usually diagnosed within six months of the occurrence of a significant stressor, and usually resolves within six months of the resolution of the stressful situation. An adjustment reaction is a short-lived anxiety response to a stressful situation. Given the time frame of this presentation, the birth and the prevalences, the most likely diagnosis is baby blues. (4, pp 285–6, 6, pp 380–1)

39. A 22-year-old man with schizophrenia, an inpatient on the psychiatric ward, develops sweating and confusion. On examination he has severe rigidity and tachycardia, and his blood pressure is fluctuating. His temperature is 106 °F. He has been treated with aripiprazole. Which of the following is the most likely diagnosis in this case?

   A. Catatonia
   B. Delirium
   C. Myocardial infarct
   D. Neuroleptic malignant syndrome
   E. Tetanus

40. A 35-year-old woman is referred to your clinic. She reports that she worked for a prominent firm but was overlooked for promotion on a number of occasions and left. She believes that others in her department conspired to prevent her promotion as they were jealous of her potential, but feels that she is overqualified for the positions available. She says that she finds it difficult to befriend women as they are often envious of her. She reports that she is currently in a wonderful relationship, which she says began two weeks previously with her new partner, an airline pilot. What is the most likely diagnosis in this case?

   A. Borderline personality disorder
   B. Histrionic personality disorder
   C. Narcissistic personality disorder
   D. Paranoid personality disorder
   E. Schizotypal personality disorder

41. A 42-year-old man presents for assessment having been transferred from another service. He tells you that he has 'manic depression'. Which of the following phenomena would most lead you to doubt this diagnosis?

   A. Delusional mood
   B. Delusional perception
   C. Delusions of persecution
   D. Flight of ideas
   E. Voices talking to the patient

42. A 48-year-old man attends for assessment. He has been transferred from another service and you have been told that he has a diagnosis of schizophrenia. Which of the following symptoms would provide the weakest evidence for this diagnosis?

   A. Delusional perception
   B. Delusions of passivity
   C. Delusions of persecution
   D. Third-person auditory hallucinations
   E. Thought broadcasting

39. Answer: D.

The diagnosis of neuroleptic malignant syndrome requires rigidity and elevated temperature in a patient on antipsychotic medication. The onset may be gradual or rapid, and most typically occurs in a young male recently commenced on neuroleptics. There are case reports in the literature of NMS occurring with aripiprazole. Catatonia may present with rigidity but is not accompanied by pyrexia or signs of autonomic instability. Tetanus presents with muscular spasm usually beginning in the masseter muscle and generalising. It is accompanied by autonomic dysfunction, but the patient is mentally alert. Delirium presents with confusion of varying degrees and may be accompanied by pyrexia though not by rigidity. Myocardial infarction may present with hypotension, diaphoresis and tachycardia, but will be marked by severe chest pain. There will be no rigidity. (10, pp 103, 106)

40. Answer: C.

This woman demonstrates the following traits of narcissistic personality disorder: has a grandiose sense of self-importance, has a sense of entitlement, believes that others are envious of her, believes that she is special and can only be understood by other special or high-status people. She has traits of other personality disorder; she including histrionic personality disorder; she considers relationships to be more intimate than they actually are. Borderline personality disorder presents with a pattern of unstable and intense interpersonal relationships. Her concern regarding her former colleagues is more a rationalisation of her failure to meet her own expectations than a pervasive distrust or suspiciousness as in a paranoid personality disorder. While she appears to lack friendships, she does not meet other criteria for a schizotypal personality disorder. (4, pp 287–97)

41. Answer: B.

Delusional perception is a first-rank symptom of schizophrenia. Delusional mood is considered not to be restricted to people with schizophrenia, but is also noted in affective disorders such as puerperal depression. (5, pp 149–54, 110)

42. Answer: C.

Delusions of persecution are a non-specific psychotic symptom. All other options are first-rank symptoms of schizophrenia. (5, pp 149–54)

43. Which of the following drugs is least likely to cause serotonin syndrome?

A. Venlafaxine
B. Ecstasy (MDMA)
C. Fluoxetine
D. Olanzapine
E. Phenelzine

44. A woman is pregnant with her first child. Her father had schizophrenia. She is afraid that her child will develop schizophrenia later in life. Which figure best represents her child's lifetime risk of developing schizophrenia?

A. 1%
B. 5%
C. 15%
D. 20%
E. 50%

45. Which of the following disorders is least likely to be an underlying cause of depressive disorder?

A. Acromegaly
B. Addison's disease
C. Cushing's disease
D. Hyperparathyroidism
E. Hypothyroidism

46. In the classification of personality disorders, which of the following disorders is contained in DSM-IV but not in ICD-10?

A. Dependent personality disorder
B. Histrionic personality disorder
C. Narcissistic personality disorder
D. Schizoid personality disorder
E. Schizotypal personality disorder

47. Which of the following personality disorders is not part of the Cluster B of personality disorders in DSM-IV?

A. Antisocial personality disorder
B. Borderline personality disorder
C. Histrionic personality disorder
D. Narcissistic personality disorder
E. Paranoid personality disorder

43. **Answer: D.**   Olanzapine is not associated with serotonin syndrome. The other drugs have all been implicated in serotonin syndrome. Ecstasy has been associated with serotonin syndrome in combination with venlafaxine. (2, pp 372–3)

44. **Answer: B.**   The grandchild of a person with schizophrenia has a 5% lifetime risk of developing the illness. The sibling of a patient where one of the parents has schizophrenia has a risk of 17%, as does the dizygotic twin of a person with schizophrenia. The monozygotic twin of a patient with schizophrenia or the child of two parents with schizophrenia has a risk of almost 50% of developing the illness. (7, p 275)

45. **Answer: A.**   Diseases of the glucocorticoid axis, Addison's and Cushing's syndromes, and of the thyroid axis may present with depressive symptoms. (3, pp 800–16)

46. **Answer: C.**   Narcissistic personality disorder is not described in the ICD-10 classification. Schizotypal disorder is listed under personality disorders in DSM-IV, but with schizophrenia in ICD-10. (11, pp 95–6, 12, p 715)

47. **Answer: E.**   Paranoid personality disorder is part of Cluster A, along with schizoid and schizotypal. The other options A–D make up Cluster B. Cluster C includes avoidant, dependent and obsessive-compulsive. (4, pp 287–97)

48. Which of the following scenarios best illustrates the defence mechanism of displacement?

    A. An overweight woman has been advised to exercise by her GP. She decides not to take exercise, as her parents, who were also both overweight, died with cardiac problems, and she thinks exercising could put undue pressure on her heart.

    B. A man who has been diagnosed with terminal cancer is belligerent and demanding with medical staff.

    C. A man who is dissatisfied with his work accuses his wife of being disappointed in him and his achievements.

    D. A woman notices a large, hard lump in her breast. She stops her regular breast examination and does not attend her GP.

    E. A woman whose mother recently died begins attending church regularly, having not attended church in a number of years. Her mother was a regular church attender.

49. A 72-year-old woman is referred for assessment by her GP. He is concerned that she is experiencing abnormal grief following the death of her husband five months previously following a long illness. Which of the following symptoms would most likely suggest that this woman is experiencing an abnormal grief reaction?

    A. Guilt

    B. Hallucinations

    C. Panic attacks

    D. Psychomotor retardation

    E. Sleep disturbance

50. Which of the following psychiatric disorders occurs with equal frequency in men and women?

    A. Agoraphobia

    B. Generalised anxiety disorder

    C. Panic disorder

    D. Simple phobia

    E. Social phobia

51. A 50-year-old man with schizophrenia is noted on examination to move his arm in response to slight pressure on it, despite being instructed to resist the pressure. Which of the following movement disorders best describes what he is exhibiting?

    A. Ambitendence

    B. Mannerism

    C. Mitgehen

    D. Stereotypy

    E. Waxy flexibility

48. Answer: B. Scenario B illustrates the defence mechanism of displacement, the transfer of emotion from a person, object or situation with which it is properly associated to a lesser source of distress. Scenario A illustrates rationalisation, the unconscious provision of a false but acceptable explanation for behaviour that has a less acceptable origin. Scenario C illustrates projection, the attribution to another person of thoughts or feelings similar to one's own thereby rendering one's own thoughts or feelings more tolerable. Scenario D illustrates denial, when a person behaves as if unaware of something that they may be reasonably expected to know. Scenario E illustrates identification, the unconscious adoption of the characteristics or activities of another person, often to reduce the pain of separation or loss. (13, p 136)

49. Answer: D. Many bereaved people experience guilt that they failed to do enough for the deceased. About one in ten will experience brief hallucinations. Sleep disturbance is very common, and anxiety may occur as panic attacks. An abnormal grief reaction occurs when the symptoms are more intense than usual and meet the criteria for a depressive disorder, if they are prolonged beyond six months, or if they are delayed in onset. This woman demonstrates many of the symptoms of normal grief; however, the symptom of psychomotor retardation is seldom present in uncomplicated grief and suggests that she is experiencing abnormally intense grief. (13, pp 152–3)

50. Answer: E. Social phobia is the only anxiety disorder to occur equally frequently in men and women. The other anxiety disorders occur approximately twice as frequently in women as in men. (13, pp 166–78)

51. Answer: C. Ambitendence occurs when the patient begins to make a movement but, before completing it starts the opposite movement, for example bending up and down over a chair without sitting on it. A mannerism is a normal, purposeful movement that appears to have social significance but is unusual in appearance. A stereotypy is a repeated purposeless movement. Waxy flexibility occurs when the patient allows himself to be placed in an awkward posture which he then maintains without distress for much longer than most people could achieve without significant discomfort. (13, pp 249–50)

52. An 18-year-old woman is referred for assessment by her GP who reports that she has lost over 20 kg in the past year. She admits that she has been restricting her diet as she believes that she is very overweight. She self-induces vomiting 2–3 times per day and has begun using laxatives. She attends the gym daily and twice on Saturday and Sunday. She has not menstruated in the last six months. Which of the following most accurately represents the biochemical profile of this woman?

A. $K^+ \downarrow$, amylase $\uparrow$, $Ca^{2+} \downarrow$, phosphate $\downarrow$
B. $K^+ \uparrow$, amylase $\uparrow$, $Ca^{2+} \downarrow$, phosphate $\downarrow$
C. $K^+ \downarrow$, amylase $\downarrow$, $Ca^{2+} \uparrow$, phosphate $\uparrow$
D. $K^+ \uparrow$, amylase $\uparrow$, $Ca^{2+} \uparrow$, phosphate $\uparrow$
E. $K^+ \uparrow$, amylase $\uparrow$, $Ca^{2+} \uparrow$, phosphate $\uparrow$

53. Which of the following psychiatric disorders has the highest lifetime risk of suicide?

A. Alcohol dependence syndrome
B. Bipolar affective disorder
C. Major depressive disorder
D. Opiate dependence
F. Schizophrenia

54. A 28-year-old man with schizophrenia reports that his wife has been replaced by a double. Which of the following syndromes is this man most likely exhibiting?

A. Capgras syndrome
B. Couvade syndrome
C. De Clerambault's syndrome
D. Fregoli's syndrome
E. Othello syndrome

55. A right-handed 72-year-old man develops right-left disorientation, finger agnosia, dyscalculia and dysgraphia. Which cerebral lobe is most likely to have been injured?

A. Left parietal lobe
B. Left temporal lobe
C. Right frontal lobe
D. Right parietal lobe
E. Right temporal lobe

56. Which of the following figures best represents the proportion of people with a mental health problem who receive their treatment in a primary care setting?

A. 5%
B. 10%
C. 20%
D. 30%
E. 50%

52. **Answer: A.** This patient has anorexia nervosa, purging type. Patients with anorexia nervosa may become hypokalemic secondary to vomiting. Amenorrhea is associated with negative calcium balance with loss of skeletal calcium in the range of 4% per year. Many eating disorder patients have significant bone mineral deficiency, usually osteopenia. Salivary amylase may be increased when purging is present. (14, pp 2014–5)

53. **Answer: B.** For bipolar affective disorder, the lifetime risk of death by suicide is 15–20%. The lifetime risk for death by suicide for the remaining options is approximately 10%. (14, pp 1184, 2447)

54. **Answer: A.** In Capgras syndrome, or delusion of doubles, the patient believes that a person known to him, usually a close relative, has been replaced by an exact double. In Fregoli's syndrome the patient believes that ordinary people in his environment are persecutors in disguise. In De Clerambault's syndrome the patient believes that another person loves him intensely. The object of the delusion is often of higher social status. In Couvade syndrome a person develops extreme anxiety and various physical symptoms of pregnancy when their partner is pregnant. Othello syndrome involves delusions of infidelity on the part of a sexual partner. (6, pp 160–3)

55. **Answer: A.** Injury of the posterior parietal lobe can result in Gerstmann's syndrome, characterised by right-left disorientation, finger agnosia (inability to recognise the fingers), dyscalculia (a defect in the ability to use mathematical symbols) and dysgraphia (disorder of writing not related to paralysis of the hands). In a right-handed person this indicates damage to the left parietal lobe. (6, p 169, 9, p 140)

56. **Answer: E.** The prevalence of diagnosable mental disorder in the general population is approximately 20% and more than one half of this group get their psychiatric care from their general practitioner. It is estimated that mental health problems constitute approximately 25% of consultations with GPs. GPs refer only 5–10% of the mental health problems they see on to a psychiatrist. (15, p 2228)

57. A 45-year-old woman with schizophrenia requires depot antipsychotic medication. She has been unsuccessfully treated with an atypical depot, and a typical depot is being considered. She has a history of third-person auditory hallucinations, persecutory delusions and depressive symptoms when unwell. Which of the following depots would be the most suitable?

A. Flupenthixol decanoate
B. Fluphenazine decanoate
C. Haloperidol decanoate
D. Pipotiazine palmitate
E. Zuclopenthixol decanoate

58. Which of the following figures best represents the proportion of patients who develop agranulocytosis on clozapine treatment?

A. 0.0001%
B. 0.1%
C. 1%
D. 5%
E. 10%

59. Which of the following antipsychotics at average daily dose has the highest monthly cost?

A. Amisulpride 800 mg daily
B. Aripiprazole 20 mg daily
C. Haloperidol 10 mg daily
D. Olanzapine 15 mg daily
E. Risperidone 6 mg daily

60. A 72-year-old woman is referred for assessment by her GP. He reports that her family have complained that she is losing her memory. He suspects that she is demonstrating features of pseudodementia rather than dementia. Which of the following features would most likely suggest that his diagnosis is correct?

A. Apraxia
B. No diurnal mood variation
C. Normal sleep/wake cycle
D. Prominent memory disturbance
E. Rapid onset

57. Answer: A. Flupenthixol decanoate is claimed to be more effective in depressed patients. Zuclopenthixol decanoate is believed to be more effective in aggressive patients, pipotiazine palmitate when EPSEs are problematic and haloperidol decanoate in the prophylaxis of manic illness. Fluphenazine decanoate is said to be associated with depressed mood. (1, p 42)

58. Answer: C. The number of patients treated with clozapine who develop agranulocytosis over one year is 0.7%. Approximately 3% of patients treated with clozapine develop neutropenia. The risk of death from clozapine-induced agranulocytosis is thought to be less than 1/10 000. (1, pp 77–8)

59. Answer: B. The proprietary costs (not including dispensing fees, or the costs attached to a private prescription) of the drugs mentioned are as follows: (1, p 18)

Amisulpride 800 mg daily	£122.76	€181.12
Aripiprazole 20 mg daily	£217.78	€321.31
Haloperidol 10 mg daily	£6.30	€8.29
Olanzapine 15 mg daily	£127.69	€188.38
Risperidone 6 mg daily	£101.01	€149.02

60. Answer: E. Patients with pseudodementia are more likely to present with rapid onset, distressed affect, fluctuating cognitive deficits, with no dyspraxia or dysphasia and a past or family history of affective disorder. Patients with dementia are more likely to present with a normal sleep/wake cycle, no diurnal variation in symptoms, gradual onset, prominent memory disturbance and focal features such as apraxia, agnosia and dysphasia; however, there can be significant overlap between dementia and pseudodementia, and patients who develop pseudodementia while depressed have a higher incidence of organic dementia at follow-up. (7, p 300)

61. A 32-year-old woman presents with multiple physical complaints for the past four years. These include headaches, abdominal pain, dysmenorrhoea, nausea, food intolerance and loss of libido. Most recently she has been complaining of difficulty swallowing, and has taken extended sick leave from work. These symptoms have been extensively investigated but no physical cause has been found. What is the most likely diagnosis in this woman's case?

A. Conversion disorder
B. Hypochondriasis
C. Major depressive episode
D. Somatisation disorder
E. Somatoform pain disorder

62. A 17-year-old male patient with a two-year history of anorexia nervosa is referred for inpatient treatment. Which of the following factors in his history will most likely worsen his prognosis?

A. Age of onset
B. Being male
C. Co-morbid depression
D. Duration of illness
E. Premorbid sexual activity

63. Which of the following individuals is most strongly associated with operant conditioning theory?

A. Bandura
B. Pavlov
C. Skinner
D. Thorndike
E. Watson

61.   Answer: D.   In somatisation disorder the patient experiences persistent recurrent multiple physical symptoms starting in early adult life or earlier. There is usually a long history of inconclusive medical and surgical investigations as well as high rates of social and occupational impairment. The DSM-IV criteria require four pain symptoms, two gastrointestinal symptoms, one sexual symptom and one pseudoneurological symptom for the diagnosis. Conversion disorder involves symptoms or deficits affecting voluntary motor or sensory function, which cannot be fully explained by a general medical condition. Hypochondriasis is distinguished from somatisation disorder by the patient's preoccupation with the underlying cause rather than symptom relief. Somatoform pain disorder is characterised by persistent severe and distressing pain at one or more anatomical sites, which is not fully explained by a physical disorder. Patients with major depressive disorder may present with non-specific physical complaints, although these do not dominate the clinical picture. In all of the above disorders, the symptoms are not intentionally produced or feigned, distinguishing them from factitious disorder or malingering. (4, pp 229–36)

62.   Answer: C.   Bad prognostic signs include psychiatric co-morbidity, very young or older age at onset and longer duration of illness. Good prognostic signs in anorexia nervosa are a short duration of illness with onset in the early to mid-teens. Male sex by itself does not confer a greater risk of a poor outcome. Men with some degree of sexual fantasy or activity before the development of anorexia nervosa have a better outcome. (14, p 2017)

63.   Answer: E.   Skinner's ideas of radical behaviourism made the effects of the environment a central feature of learning. Operant conditioning is a form of learning in which behavioural frequency is altered through the application of positive and negative consequences. Thorndike preceded Skinner in identifying the relationship between appropriate behaviour and experiences of success and failure. Pavlov and Watson are associated with classical conditioning, the association of a neutral stimulus with an unconditioned stimulus such that the neutral stimulus comes to bring about a response similar to that originally elicited by the unconditioned stimulus. Pavlov performed experiments examining the idea that learning occurs when two events occur closely together. Watson demonstrated that classical conditioning can give rise to phobia-like behaviour in a famous experiment involving an 11-month-old infant, in which he paired a loud noise with the sight of a white rat, leading the child to fear the rat and also similar objects, an example of stimulus generalisation. Bandura advocated social cognitive learning theory, which argues that the influence of environmental events on the acquisition and the regulation of behaviour is primarily a function of cognitive processes. (15, pp 541–7)

64. A 32-year-old man presents following a road traffic accident six months previously in which he was severely injured. He experiences recurrent nightmares of the event and distressing intrusive memories. He does not drive and avoids the area in which the accident occurred. What form of learning most likely contributes to the avoidance symptoms exhibited by this patient?

A. Classical conditioning
B. Instrumental learning
C. Modelling
D. Operant conditioning
E. Social-cognitive learning

65. A 20-year-old woman experiences episodes in which she falls down with a sudden loss of muscle tone after which she sleeps. These episodes tend to be provoked by strong emotion. What symptom best describes what this woman is experiencing?

A. Catalepsy
B. Cataplexy
C. Catatonia
D. Cathexis
E. Sleep paralysis

66. An inpatient with schizoaffective disorder says the following 'the man in the van, can, can. He's a plan to stand, understand. The band fanned me.' What form of language disorder is he most likely exhibiting?

A. Clang association
B. Echopraxia
C. Metonymy
D. Palilalia
E. Verbigeration

67. Which of the following brain structures is least likely included in the limbic system?

A. Amygdala
B. Hippocampal formation
C. Hypothalamus
D. Parahippocampal cingulate gyrus
E. Posterior nucleus of the thalamus

68. Which of the following patients carries the most risk factors for tardive dyskinesia?

A. A male patient with schizophrenia who has never taken antipsychotic medications.
B. A young female patient with bipolar disorder.
C. An elderly female patient with bipolar disorder.
D. An elderly female patient with schizophrenia.
E. An elderly male patient with schizoaffective disorder.

64. Answer: A. Classical conditioning explains how stimuli associated with a severe trauma come to elicit stress responses that were part of the original trauma. Instrumental learning is another term for operant conditioning. Modelling is observational learning. Social-cognitive theory espouses the influence of environmental events on the acquisition, and the regulation of behaviour is primarily a function of cognitive processes. (15, pp 541–7)

65. Answer: B. Cataplexy is temporary sudden loss of muscle tone, causing weakness and immobilisation. It can be precipitated by a variety of emotional states and is often followed by sleep. It is commonly seen in narcolepsy. Catalepsy is a condition in which a person maintains the body position in which they are placed. It is seen in catatonic schizophrenia and is also called waxy flexibility. Cathexis is a term from psychoanalysis meaning a conscious or unconscious investment of psychic energy into an idea, concept, object or person. Sleep paralysis is an episode of inability to move occurring between wakefulness and sleep, in either direction. Catatonic stupor is a state of decreased reactivity to stimuli in which the patient is aware of their surroundings. (5, p 43, 14, pp 849–59)

66. Answer: A. A clang association is the association of speech directed by the sound of a word rather than by its meaning. It includes punning and rhyming speech and is most often seen in schizophrenia and mania. It has been suggested that the clang associations in the language disorder of schizophrenia involve the initial syllable of a previous word, while the clang in manic speech occurs in terminal syllables. Echolalia is the repeating of words or phrases of one person by another. It is particularly seen in catatonic schizophrenia. Metonymy involves the use of a word or phrase that is related to the proper one but not the one ordinarily used; for example the patient says he will eat a menu rather than a meal. Palilalia is the repetition of a word or phrase. It is a perseveratory phenomenon. Verbigeration is the meaningless and stereotyped repetition of words or phrases seen in schizophrenia. (5, p 167, 14, pp 849–59)

67. Answer: E. The limbic system includes the anterior nucleus of the thalamus. Different authorities list different components, but generally the limbic system includes the hippocampus, mammillary bodies, hypothalamus, anterior nucleus of the thalamus, septal nuclei, fornix, cingulate gyrus, parahippocampal gyrus, amygdala, nucleus accumbens and the mammillothalamic tract. (7, p 24)

68. Answer: C. Although tardive dyskinesia can occur in patients who have never taken antipsychotics, it is much more common in those who have taken antipsychotic drugs for many years. Tardive dyskinesia is more common among women, the elderly and those with diffuse brain pathology. A diagnosis of an affective disorder is also a risk factor. (6, p 316)

69. For which of the following antipsychotic side effects are anticholinergic drugs least suitable?

    A. Akathisia
    B. Dystonia
    C. Rigidity
    D. Tardive dyskinesia
    E. Tremor

70. A 35-year-old married woman is referred for assessment by her GP who reports that she is having sexual difficulties. She is physically well. The patient reports that she and her husband both enjoy an intimate relationship but have been unable to achieve penetration. Which of the following is the most likely diagnosis?

    A. Female orgasmic disorder
    B. Female sexual arousal disorder
    C. Hypoactive sexual desire disorder
    D. Sexual aversion disorder
    E. Vaginismus

71. A 55-year-old patient being treated for depressive disorder has shown very little response to medication. Which of the following factors would be the strongest predictor of this man's positive response to electroconvulsive therapy?

    A. Delusions
    B. Hypochondriacal symptoms
    C. Personality disorder
    D. Previous response to electroconvulsive therapy
    E. Psychomotor retardation

72. Which of the following is least likely to be an indication for electroconvulsive therapy?

    A. Mania
    B. Neuroleptic malignant syndrome
    C. Obsessive compulsive disorder
    D. Parkinson's disease
    E. Schizophrenia

73. Which of the following features is least likely a characteristic of a hypnotic state?

    A. Acceptance of distortions
    B. Attention is indiscriminately directed
    C. Diminished reality testing
    D. Increased suggestibility
    E. Post-hypnotic amnesia

69. Answer: D.

The appropriate treatment for tardive dyskinesia is slow withdrawal or reduction in antipsychotic medication, and consideration of an alternative. Anticholinergic medications can provoke or exacerbate tardive dyskinesia. Anticholinergics are an appropriate treatment option for antipsychotic-induced tremor, dystonia and rigidity. Anticholinergics may have some efficacy in treating akathisia, which is part of an extra pyramidal side-effect profile. (2, pp 97–104)

70. Answer: E.

Sexual disorders can be categorised into those affecting sexual desire, affecting sexual arousal, affecting orgasm and causing pain. Vaginismus is a recurrent or persistent involuntary spasm of the musculature of the outer third of the vagina that interferes with sexual intercourse. It is the only one of the female sexual disorders that prevents completion of sexual intercourse. (4, pp 245–50, 13, pp 488–90)

71. Answer: D.

Hypochondriasis and personality disorder are two negative predictors of response to ECT. Psychomotor retardation and delusions are positive predictors; however a history of previous response to ECT is the most robust predictor of all. (7, pp 602–3)

72. Answer: C.

An acute response to ECT has been demonstrated in OCD, but patients soon relapsed and ECT is not recommended for this disorder. The use of ECT in mania is reserved for patients who are resistant or intolerant to the usual medication treatments or who have severe symptoms, for example manic delirium. Neuorleptic malignant syndrome shows outcomes with ECT which are equivalent to those obtained pharmacologically. Schizophrenia is the second most common indication for ECT, although there is a lack of consensus about its use in this disorder. Motor symptoms in Parkinson's disease have been shown to be lessened by ECT, with effects lasting 4–6 weeks. (14, pp 2972–4)

73. Answer: B.

The characteristics of a hypnotic state have been described as follows: the subject ceases to make his own plans. Attention is selectively directed, for example towards the voice of the hypnotist. Reality testing is decreased and distortions are accepted. Suggestibility is increased. The subject readily enacts unusual roles. Post-hypnotic amnesia is often present. (5, p 47)

74. A 35-year-old man with schizophrenia reports that he has realised that he is being targeted by a terrorist organisation that is accessing his thoughts through the Internet. When asked what makes him think this he replies that he does not 'think' it, but that it is true. He says that the realisation came to him 'out of the blue'. Which of the following options best describes this man's experience?

A. Autochthonous delusion
B. Delusional memory
C. Delusional mood
D. Delusional percept
E. Nihilistic delusions

75. A patient with schizophrenia shows marked disturbance of speech. While the words he uses are recognisable they are so disorganised in sentences that they are meaningless. Which of the following speech disorders best describes this speech disturbance?

A. Cluttering
B. Echolalia
C. Logoclonia
D. Palilalia
E. Paragrammatism

76. Which of the following medications acts primarily by modifying serotonin degradation?

A. Clomipramine
B. Fluoxetine
C. Mirtazapine
D. Phenelzine
E. Venlafaxine

77. A 55-year-old woman with a history of depressive disorder tells you that she is planning to go out for a meal to celebrate her birthday. She is currently taking phenelzine. Which of the following foods is safest for this woman to order?

A. Brie cheese
B. Caviar
C. Guacamole
D. Pheasant
E. Fresh sausages

74. Answer: A.

The patient is describing an autochthonous delusion or delusional intuition, which occurs out of the blue to the patient. Delusional intuition occurs in one stage, unlike a delusional percept that occurs in two stages: perception followed by false interpretation. Delusional mood refers to a feeling of anticipation that something significant is going to happen. The patient feels perplexed, apprehensive and uncomfortable. It is followed by the formation of a delusion and tends to occur in the early development of a schizophrenic illness. Delusional memory occurs when the patient recounts as remembered an event or idea that is delusional in nature. It has the characteristics of a delusional percept or delusional intuition but is remembered from the past rather than in the present. These terms all refer to the form of the delusion. Nihilistic refers to the content of the delusion and describes an extremely negative belief. (5, pp 104–11, 121)

75. Answer: E.

Paragrammatism refers to the disorder of grammatical construction. In schizophrenia it is termed *word salad*. Cluttering is a disturbance of fluency involving an abnormally rapid rate and erratic rhythm of speech that impedes intelligibility. In echolalia the patient repeats words or parts of sentences that are spoken to him or in his presence. It most often occurs in excited schizophrenic states, with learning disability and with organic states. Logoclonia describes the spastic repetition of syllables that occurs in Parkinsonism. Palilalia is the repetition of a word or phrase. It is a perseveratory phenomenon. (5, pp 158–9, 14, pp 849–59)

76. Answer: D.

Phenelzine is a monoamine oxidase inhibitor. Monamine oxidase oxidises most serotonin to 5-hydroxyindoleacetaldehyde. It is then broken down to 5-hydroxyindoleacetic acid (5-HIAA) by aldehyde dehydrogenase, the major metabolite of serotonin degradation. Fluoxetine acts as a selective serotonin reuptake inhibitor. Clomipramine inhibits the reuptake of serotonin, and its metabolite desmethylclomipramine inhibits the reuptake of noradrenaline. Mirtazapine is a noradrenergic and specific serotonergic antidepressant that acts by inhibiting α-2 receptors to specifically increase serotonin at the 5HT1A receptor and increase noradrenergic transmission. Venlafaxine is a serotonin and noradrenaline reuptake inhibitor at medium-to-high doses. (8, pp 62–74, 420)

77. Answer: E.

When taking MAOIs it is important to avoid tyramine-containing foods because of the risk of hypertensive crisis. The patient must also avoid foods that are matured or may be spoiling. Soft mature cheeses, guacamole and caviar all contain levels of tyramine, which should be avoided. Pheasant is a game fowl that is hung and may be spoiled. Fresh sausages have been found to contain only minute amounts of tyramine and are not considered a particular risk (dry cured sausages have higher levels of tyramine). (2, pp 300–1)

78. A 22-year-old woman working as an administrative manager is referred by her GP who reports that she is suicidal. She is accompanied by her parents with whom she has a good relationship. The patient tells you that she has been feeling depressed for about three months and has been feeling worse in the last two weeks. She has never harmed herself in the past. Which of this patient's characteristics would most likely increase your concern regarding her suicidal risk?

   A. Employment status
   B. Gender
   C. Socioeconomic group
   D. Mental illness
   E. Social support

79. A 44-year-old man is diagnosed by his GP with a depressive disorder. He is commenced on escitalopram 10 mg daily. After six weeks he has shown no response to treatment. Which of the following is the most appropriate next step?

   A. Add bupropion
   B. Add lithium
   C. Change to an alternative antidepressant
   D. Consider electroconvulsant therapy
   E. Increase the dose of escitalopram

80. A 45-year-old woman attending your service has been diagnosed with a depressive disorder. However, she has shown little response to her antidepressant medication. She has been on escitalopram 5 mg for six weeks with no response. She complains of loss of libido since commencing on the medication. She is also taking cimetidine. What is the likely cause of treatment resistance in this woman's case?

   A. Drug interactions
   B. Inadequate dosage of antidepressant
   C. Insufficient time for antidepressant to be effective
   D. Non-compliance
   E. Unaddressed psychiatric comorbidity

81. A 55-year-old man has a long history of schizophrenia. He has a disorganisation syndrome, characterised by inappropriate affect, poverty of content of speech, tangentiality, derailment and distractability. This symptom cluster was best described by which of the following researchers?

   A. Andreasen
   B. Bleuler
   C. Crowe
   D. Liddle
   E. Schneider

78. Answer: D.   The factors for increased risk of suicide include male gender, lack of social support, unemployment, lower socioeconomic category, especially for those in a middle age group, severe mental illness, especially depression and a history of self-harm. This woman's mental illness is her most significant risk factor. (16, p 400)

79. Answer: E.   If the patient fails to respond to the average dose of an antidepressant, provided he is tolerating the medication, he should first be prescribed a higher dose. If there is still no improvement in a further two weeks then an alternative antidepressant should be considered. If following an adequate trial of the alternative antidepressant at an adequate dose he still shows no improvement then treatments for refractory depression should be considered. (1, p 187)

80. Answer: B.   This woman has been taking only 5 mg escitalopram, albeit for an adequate period of six weeks. The recommended dose for the treatment of depression is 10 mg daily, increasing to a maximum of 20 mg. Loss of libido is a potential side effect of escitalopram indicating that this patient is compliant with her medication. Escitalopram has a low likelihood of drug interaction, so the co-prescription of cimetidine is unlikely to be causing a difficulty. (2, pp 54, 279)

81. Answer: D.   Liddle described three syndromes of chronic schizophrenia: psychomotor poverty syndrome, disorganisation syndrome and reality distortion syndrome. Andreasen divided schizophrenia into two syndromes, positive and negative, according to a set of validated diagnostic criteria. Crowe described Type I and Type II syndromes on the basis of post-mortem findings. Subsequent research evidence showed that cognitive impairment and tardive dyskinesia occur most commonly in patients with Type II syndrome and are infrequent in those with Type 1 schizophrenia. Bleuler is known for describing the primary or fundamental symptoms of schizophrenia as the 'four As': autism, ambivalence, abnormal association and affective abnormality. Schneider described the first-rank symptoms of schizophrenia, which he believed differentiated schizophrenia from similar illnesses. (7, pp 259–60, 266–7)

82. A 35-year-old woman is referred for assessment by her GP who reports that she has been complaining of widespread pain for the last five months. She has complained of pain in various areas on both the right and left sides of her body, above and below the waist. She additionally complains of fatigue, low mood and sleep disturbance. On examination she exhibits tenderness in many areas, including the occiput, trapezius, gluteus and knees. Physical investigations are normal. What is the most likely diagnosis in this woman's case?

   A. Body dysmorphic disorder
   B. Fibromyalgia
   C. Hypochondriasis
   D. Rheumatoid arthritis
   E. Somatisation disorder

83. A 45-year-old Asian man is referred by his GP for assessment. He recently arrived in the country and is concerned that his penis is shrinking. On further interview the patient expresses the fear that his penis will eventually disappear into his body and that he will then die. He has marked anxiety symptoms. His family report that he has tied a string to his penis in an attempt to stop the perceived shrinking. Which of the following culture-bound syndromes is this patient most likely experiencing?

   A. Amok
   B. Brain fag
   C. *Dhat*
   D. Koro
   E. Latah

82.   Answer: B.

The primary symptom of fibromyalgia is widespread pain with tenderness at multiple specified anatomical sites for at least three months. The most common associated symptoms are fatigue, depression, sleep disturbances and cognitive problems. Depression and anxiety often develop and exacerbate the condition. Body dysmorphic disorder involves preoccupation with an imagined defect in appearance. Hypochondriasis is characterised by preoccupation with fears of having, or the idea that one has, a serious disease based on the misinterpretation of bodily symptoms. The duration of disturbance is at least six months. In somatisation disorder the patient experiences persistent recurrent multiple physical symptoms starting in early adult life or earlier. There is usually a long history of inconclusive investigations and procedures, and high rates of social and occupational impairment. The DSM-IV criteria require four pain symptoms, two gastrointestinal symptoms, one sexual symptom, and one pseudoneurological symptom for the diagnosis. The diagnosis of rheumatoid arthritis will be assisted by the presence of morning stiffness, symmetrical arthritis at multiple joints and the presence of rheumatoid nodules. Positive rheumatoid factor is present in about 80%, and there may also be changes on X-ray. (4, pp 229–36, 17, p 2178)

83.   Answer: D.

Koro involves an episode of sudden and intense anxiety that the penis will recede into the body and possibly cause death. It is associated with a feeling of overwhelming panic. The patient may attempt to prevent retraction. The syndrome is reported in South and East Asia. *Dhat* is a term used in India to refer to severe anxiety and hypochondriacal concerns associated with the discharge of semen, whitish discoloration of the urine, and feelings of weakness and exhaustion. Latah is hypersensitivity to sudden fright, often with echopraxia, echolalia, command obedience and dissociative behaviour. The syndrome has been found in many parts of the world. Brain fag is a term initially used in West Africa to refer to a condition experienced by student in response to the challenges of schooling. Symptoms include difficulties in concentrating, remembering and thinking. Amok is a dissociative episode characterised by a period of brooding followed by an outburst of violent aggressive or homicidal behaviour directed at people and objects. (14, pp 2286–9)

84. A patient with epilepsy reports frequent seizures. He initially experiences an intense fear, followed by a period of absence, amnesia and motor activity. He is confused following the seizure. Which term best describes this seizure?

   A. Petit-mal
   B. Complex-partial
   C. Partial seizures evolving to secondarily generalised seizures
   D. Simple-partial
   E. Tonic-clonic

85. A 55-year-old patient who has been drinking alcohol heavily for over ten years attends the service requesting information about alcohol support services. What stage of the change cycle is this patient most likely at?

   A. Action
   B. Contemplation
   C. Decision
   D. Maintenance
   E. Precontemplation

84. Answer: B.

Generalised seizures involve abnormal electrical activity, which is widespread in the brain and results in loss of consciousness. Partial seizures involve abnormal electrical activity in a focal area of the brain, which may or may not result in loss of consciousness. A partial seizure may evolve into a generalised seizure. Simple-partial seizures usually have an abrupt onset and ending and last only a few seconds, with no loss of consciousness. Complex-partial seizures are the most common type of partial seizures. They are characterised by the presence of an aura, followed by a period of absence, amnesia, loss of consciousness and motor activity. They may be accompanied by an automatism. Tonic-clonic seizures are generalised seizures involving loss of consciousness and a tonic phase during which there is sudden spasm of all the muscles of the body for several seconds. This is followed by rhythmic jerking of the limbs and head, the clonic phase. Petit-mal seizures are generalised seizures characterised by loss of awareness of one's surroundings. The attack last a few seconds and consciousness is lost. (8, pp 315–6)

85. Answer: C.

The cycle of change proposed by Prochaska and DiClemente, originally developed to describe the process people go through in giving up smoking, is also applied to drinking behaviour. The stages are as follows:

Precontemplation: The person does not see any harm in their behaviour.

Contemplation: The person is unsure whether they want to change their behaviour or not.

Decision/Determination: The person has decided to do something and is getting ready for change.

Action: The person has made the change.

Maintenance: The change has been integrated into the person's life.

Relapse: There is full return of the old behaviour.

The man in the question has decided to change and is preparing to do so by seeking support. (7, pp 237–8)

86. An EEG shows high-voltage slow waves all over the scalp. δ Waves account for <50% of the rhythm. Sleep spindles and K complexes diminish. What stage of the sleep cycle is the EEG most likely detecting?

   A. Stage I
   B. Stage II
   C. Stage III
   D. Stage IV
   E. Wakefulness

87. A 25-year-old man with schizophrenia tells you that thoughts are being taken out of his head by terrorists. He says that these terrorists are responsible for transmitting his thoughts to others, who use his words to write songs. What form of thought disorder is this man experiencing?

   A. Audible thoughts
   B. Thought blocking
   C. Thought broadcasting
   D. Thought insertion
   E. Thought withdrawal

88. A 55-year-old patient with a history of alcohol dependence is admitted to the hospital for alcohol detoxification. He is noted on assessment to have clouding of consciousness. On physical examination, he is found to have paralysis of the external rectus muscle, paralysis of conjugate gaze, ataxia and peripheral polyneuropathy. Ophthalmoscopic examination reveals retinal haemorrhages. What vitamin deficiency is most likely responsible for this clinical picture?

   A. A
   B. B_1
   C. B_{12}
   D. E
   E. K

89. A 44-year-old man is referred for assessment by his GP who reports that he has been complaining of memory loss following a road traffic accident. Which of the following findings would most likely suggest that this man is malingering?

   A. Dense anterograde amnesia
   B. Loss of consciousness at the time of the accident
   C. Performance worse than chance level on neuropsychological testing
   D. Perseveration
   E. Retrograde amnesia

86. Answer: C.

The EEG features of sleep may be summarised as follows:

Stage I: The occipital α rhythm slowly disappears, and low-voltage desynchronised slow waves (θ and δ) appear.

Stage II: Low voltages and δ and slower frequencies dominate the recording. Sleep spindles and K complexes occur.

Stage III: High-voltage slow waves occur all over the scalp. δ Waves account for <50% of the rhythm. Sleep spindles and K complexes diminish.

Stage IV: δ Waves dominate the EEG accounting for >50% of the rhythm. Sleep spindles and K complexes are absent.

Wakefulness: Characterised by the high-frequency β rhythm.
(7, p 536)

87. Answer: B.

Option B is a disorder of thought form. Option A is a type of auditory hallucination. The remaining options are delusions, or disorders of thought content. Thought blocking is a form of thought disorder in which the patient experiences his chain of thoughts snapping off or stopping unexpectedly. This patient interprets this experience as a delusion of thought control. He believes that his thoughts are being taken out of his head by another agency (thought withdrawal). In an additional delusion of thought control, he also believes that his thoughts are being dispersed widely out of his control (thought broadcasting). Thought insertion is a third delusion of thought control, in which the patient believes that thoughts are being inserted into his head. This is a delusional interpretation of the thought disorder. Audible thoughts in which a patient hears their own thoughts out loud are a form of auditory hallucination. (5, pp 140–1,148)

88. Answer: C.

This patient has developed Wernicke's encephalopathy as a result of vitamin B_{12} or thiamine deficiency. He is likely to be deficient in all vitamins as a result of malnutrition. (8, p 1105)

89. Answer: C.

The diagnosis of malingering is made when the features of the presentation and history are atypical for an amnestic disorder. The patient may feign amnesia in preparation for legal proceedings. On neuropsychological testing a pattern of performance that is worse than chance or guessing suggests manipulation of the results for deliberate failure. Densely amnestic patients score at least at a chance level of 50% accuracy simply by guessing. Malingering patients may purposely avoid the correct response and score below chance. On tests of progressive difficulty, the malingering patient might perform poorly even on the easier tasks and may not demonstrate the graduated decrements in performance of an amnestic patient. The remaining options are suggestive of a true amnesia. (8, p 1105)

90. A man who believes in the rights of the disabled finds that there is no parking space beside his workplace. It is raining heavily and he is late for an important meeting. There are two parking spaces for the disabled available. He parks in a disabled parking space. Which of the following factors will most likely decrease his cognitive dissonance?

    A. A sign requesting that drivers refrain from using the disabled parking spaces.
    B. Deciding that disabled parking spaces discriminate against drivers without a disability.
    C. The approach of a traffic warden.
    D. The knowledge that there are parking spaces five minutes' walk away.
    E. The knowledge that two of his co-workers are disabled.

91. A 40-year-old patient with a history of alcohol dependence syndrome is currently abstinent from alcohol. He reports that he feels ready to return to work. Which of the following features of this man's plans for employment would least concern you?

    A. Autonomous working
    B. Mobility
    C. Office environment
    D. Sale of alcohol
    E. Spending much time away from home

92. A patient with bipolar affective disorder on lithium therapy complains of sudden onset of tremor. His speech is slurred at interview, and his gait is unsteady. His serum lithium is 2.0 mmol/L. Which of the following is most likely to have contributed to the development of lithium toxicity?

    A. Alcohol
    B. Caffeine
    C. Frusemide
    D. Lamotrigine
    E. Warfarin

93. A 54-year-old woman is due to have electroconvulsive therapy for the treatment of a severe depressive episode. She is reluctant as she has heard that it can cause severe memory problems. What type of memory difficulty is this patient most likely to experience?

    A. Immediate memory impairment
    B. Long-term permanent anterograde amnesia
    C. Retrograde amnesia for remote events
    D. Short-term anterograde amnesia
    E. Short-term retrograde amnesia

90. **Answer: B.** Cognitive dissonance theory, proposed by Festinger in 1957, suggests that individuals strive for consistency in their attitudes, with discomfort or dissonance arising if two cognitions are held that are inconsistent. Dissonance is increased by low pressure to comply, increased choice of options, awareness of responsibility for consequences, expectation of unpleasant consequences of behaviour towards others. Dissonance is decreased by changing behaviour, dismissing information, adding new cognitions. This man decreases his dissonance by changing his attitudes towards the rights of the disabled. (7, p 93)

91. **Answer: C.** The factors that increase the risk of relapse in the work environment are job mobility, an absence of the restraining structure of home/regular workplace, the absence of supervision at work, and the ready availability of alcohol. (6, p 121)

92. **Answer: C.** Thiazide diuretics reduce the renal clearance of lithium and levels can rise within a few days. Excessive caffeine can cause a decrease in lithium levels. A rapid decrease in caffeine intake can result in lithium toxicity. Alcohol may result in a slight increase (about 12%) in peak lithium levels. There is no documented interaction between lithium and lamotrigine or warfarin. (2, pp 302–6)

93. **Answer: D.** Most patients will experience some degree of anterograde amnesia, particularly if the patient is confused after the treatment. Some patients will have difficult retaining new learning for a few days or even weeks after a course of ECT. This impairment, while common, is short-lived. A smaller number of patients will experience a retrograde amnesia for events leading up to and during a course of ECT. Some patients will report holes or gaps in their memory extending back several years. The issue of long-term permanent anterograde amnesia is unresolved but is complained of only by a minority. Immediate memory refers to the sensory store in which information is held for less than a second in the form in which it was perceived. This level is not usually affected in organic memory disorders. (5, p 49, 8, pp 894–6)

94. A patient is admitted to a psychiatric hospital as a voluntary patient. During his admission he tells his doctor that he no longer wishes to take medication. His doctor tells him that if he does not take medication his status will be changed to involuntary and he will be given medication by force. What ethical principle has this doctor most transgressed?

A. Autonomy
B. Beneficence
C. Justice
D. Non-maleficence
E. Confidentiality

95. A 35-year-old male patient with schizophrenia and a history of violence when unwell reports that he has stopped taking his medication as he was experiencing intolerable side effects. He has been thinking about killing his psychiatrist, who he blames for the breakdown of his marriage, and expresses a number of delusional beliefs about his ex-wife's fidelity. A decision is taken to admit the man as an involuntary patient. Which of the following best represents the ethical tension that this scenario presents?

A. Autonomy vs. Beneficence
B. Autonomy vs. Non-maleficence
C. Beneficence vs. Justice
D. Beneficence vs. Non-maleficence
E. Non-maleficence vs. Justice

96. A 36-year-old man with an episode of severe depression, unresponsive to antidepressant therapy, is undergoing a course of ECT. On his first treatment, despite two applications of an electrical stimulus, the fit is of sub-maximal duration. Which of the following medications is most likely to be causing the difficulty?

A. Chlorpromazine
B. Clomipramine
C. Diazepam
D. Lithium
E. Phenelzine

97. Which of the following disorders typically has the oldest age at onset?

A. Anorexia nervosa
B. Asperger's syndrome
C. Gilles de la Tourette's syndrome
D. Obsessive compulsive disorder
E. Social phobia

94. Answer: A.

The four main ethical principles of medical treatment are:

Autonomy: Respecting the freedom of the patient to make choices regarding their treatment

Beneficence: Placing the benefit to the patient at the forefront of clinical practice

Non-maleficence: Doing no harm

Justice: This refers to both individual and social justice.

This doctor has adopted a coercive approach to treatment. While one might argue that this does harm to the patient, and certainly to the therapeutic relationship, it most clearly compromises the patient's autonomy. (18, pp 41–4)

95. Answer: A.

The four main ethical principles of medical treatment as outlined above are: Autonomy, Beneficence, Non-maleficence and Justice. In this scenario, the patient's right to make choices about his treatment is in conflict with the doctor's obligation to do good for the patient. Given the stated intent to harm a specified person, the psychiatrist is most likely to treat the patient against his will overruling his autonomy. This scenario might also be represented by a tension between autonomy and justice, considering the doctor's duty to protect third parties. (18, pp 41–4)

96. Answer: C.

Benzodiazepines are likely to raise the seizure threshold, reduce seizure duration and increase the number of treatments needed. Lithium used with ECT is reported to result in severe memory difficulties, neurological difficulties and a reduced antidepressant effect. Owing to the additional potential for ECT to result in lithium toxicity, this combination should be used only with very clear indications. MAOIs are normally contraindicated with anaesthetics as they can interact with opiates, but there is thought to be no significant problem with ECT itself. Tricyclics and ECT combined are thought to produce few difficulties, although the combinations with anaesthetic agents may raise the risk of cardiac arrhythmias and hypotension. Antipsychotics lower the seizure threshold and would be expected to lead to seizures at lower ECT doses. (2, pp 158–60)

97. Answer: D.

The mean age of onset for obsessive compulsive disorder is 20 years. Social phobia typically begins to develop after puberty. The mean age of onset of Gilles de la Tourette's syndrome is seven years. Features of Asperger's syndrome are commonly noted from the age of three or earlier. The majority of females with anorexia nervosa have onset within five year of menarche. (6, pp 68, 75, 93, 277, 287)

98. A baby and his carer enter an unfamiliar room. A stranger enters and the carer leaves. The baby's play decreases and he appears upset. When the carer returns he greets her, stays close to her and begins to re-explore. According to Ainsworth what type of attachment is this baby most likely displaying?

A. Autonomous
B. Disorganised
C. Insecure-ambivalent
D. Insecure-avoidant
E. Secure attachment

99. A 45-year-old patient with schizophrenia is unemployed and lives with his mother. Attempts have been made to engage him in an occupational therapy programme, but he shows poor motivation. He was last hospitalised about two years ago when he had persecutory delusions, delusions of reference and second- and third-party auditory hallucinations. More recently he appears to harbour the same delusions but is not preoccupied by them. He reports that he occasionally hears voices but they do not bother him. According to DSM-IV, what type of schizophrenia best describes this man's symptoms?

A. Catatonic
B. Disorganised
C. Paranoid
D. Residual
E. Undifferentiated

100. A 40-year-old man is referred for assessment. While taking his history you note that he expresses a lot of anger towards his parents and is preoccupied with events from his childhood. According to Main, which form of adult attachment is this man most likely to display?

A. Autonomous
B. Dismissing
C. Disorganised
D. Preoccupied
E. Unresolved

98. Answer: E.

Sixty to seventy per cent of infants show secure attachment. Insecure-avoidant infants do not appear upset as the mother leaves. On her return they stay close to her but avoid her if picked up (20%). Infants with an insecure-ambivalent attachment appear upset when left, but are ambivalent on her return, reaching out but pushing her away at the same time (10%). Infants in the disorganised attachment category lack consistency in their behaviour (10–15%). Autonomous is a form of adult attachment that has been linked to childhood secure attachment. (7, p 66)

99. Answer: D.

Residual schizophrenia involves an absence of prominent delusions, hallucinations, disorganised speech, or grossly disorganised or catatonic behaviour. There is continuing evidence of disturbance with negative symptoms or two or more positive symptoms present in attenuated form. In disorganised schizophrenia disorganised speech, disorganised behaviour and a flat or inappropriate affect are prominent. Catatonic schizophrenia is characterised by at least two of the following: motor immobility, excessive motor activity, extreme negativism, peculiarities of voluntary movement, of echolalia or echopraxia. Paranoid schizophrenia involves a preoccupation with one or more delusions or frequent auditory hallucinations. Undifferentiated schizophrenia meets the core criteria for schizophrenia but criteria for the other subtypes are not met. (4, pp 155–7)

100. Answer: D.

Preoccupied attachment has been linked to insecure-ambivalent attachment in childhood. Adults displaying autonomous attachment are self-reliant, coherent in describing early experiences, objective and not defensive. It has been linked with secure attachment in childhood. Adults with a dismissing pattern of attachment appear to have few emotional memories of childhood. They tend to idealise cares and minimise the effects of traumatic events. This is thought to correspond to an insecure-avoidant attachment pattern in childhood. Adults with a pattern of unresolved attachment display gaps in their account of childhood, particularly around traumatic events. This has been linked with disorganised childhood attachment. (7, p 67)

References

1. Taylor D, Paton C, Kerwin R. *The South London and Maudsley NHS Foundation Trust and Oxleas NHS Foundation Trust: prescribing guidelines*. 9th ed. London: Informa Healthcare; 2007.
2. Bazire S. *Psychotropic Drug Directory 2005: the professionals' pocket handbook and aide memoire*. Salisbury: Fivepin; 2005.
3. Kumar P, Clark M. *Clinical Medicine: a textbook for medical students and doctors*. London; Philadelphia, PA: Baillière Tindall; 1994.
4. American Psychiatric Association. *Desk Reference to the Diagnostic Criteria from DSM-IV-TR*. Washington, DC: American Psychiatric Association; 2000.
5. Sims A. *Symptoms in the Mind: an introduction to descriptive psychopathology*. 2nd ed. London: Saunders; 1995.
6. Buckley P, Bird J, Harrison G. *Examination Notes in Psychiatry: a postgraduate text*. Oxford: Butterworth-Heinemann; 1995.
7. Wright P, Stern J, Phelan M. *Core Psychiatry*. London: WB Saunders; 2000.
8. Freeman CPL, Zealley AK. *Companion to Psychiatric Studies*. 6th ed. Johnstone EC, editor. Edinburgh: Churchill Livingstone; 1998.
9. Bannister R. *Brain's Clinical Neurology*. London; New York: Oxford University Press; 1985.
10. Taylor D, Paton C, Kerwin R, editors. *The Maudsley Prescribing Guidelines*. 9th ed. London: Informa Healthcare; 2007.
11. World Health Organization. *The ICD-10 Classification of Mental and Behavioural Disorders: clinical descriptions and diagnostic guidelines*. Geneva: World Health Organization; 1992.
12. American Psychiatric Association. *Diagnostic and Statistical Manual of Mental Disorders: DSM-IV-TR*. Washington, DC: American Psychiatric Association; 2000.
13. Gelder MG, Gath D, Mayou R. *Oxford Textbook of Psychiatry*. 3rd ed. Oxford; New York: Oxford University Press; 1996.
14. Sadock BJ, Sadock VA, Kaplan HI. *Kaplan & Sadock's Comprehensive Textbook of Psychiatry*. 8th ed. Philadelphia, PA: Lippincott Williams & Wilkins; 2005.
15. Sadock B, Sadock V. *Kaplan & Sadock's Comprehensive Textbook of Psychiatry*. 7th ed. Philadelphia, PA: Lippincott Williams & Wilkins; 2000.
16. Puri BK, Hall AD. *Revision Notes in Psychiatry*. 2nd ed. London: Arnold; 2004.
17. Kaplan HI, Sadock BJ. *Comprehensive Textbook of Psychiatry*. 6 ed. Baltimore, MD: Lippincott Williams & Wilkins; 1995.
18. Mills S. *Clinical Practice and the Law*: Dublin: Tottel; 2002.

chapter 02

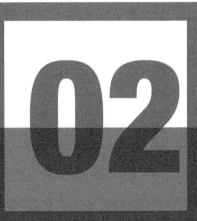

100 MCQs from Dr. Guy Molyneaux and Colleagues

Dr Pauline Devitt; Dr Angela Noonan; Dr Klaus Oliver Schubert; and Prof Finian O'Brien

101. Which one of the following psychotropic drugs has the shortest elimination half-life ($t_{1/2}$)?

A. Haloperidol
B. Lithium
C. Trazodone
D. Tranylcypromine
E. Chlormethiazole

102. Which one of the following antidepressants has non-linear pharmacokinetic properties?

A. Citalopram
B. Fluoxetine
C. Escitalopram
D. Sertraline
E. Amfebutamone (bupropion)

103. Which of the following benzodiazepines has the shortest elimination half-life ($t_{1/2}$)?

A. Lorazepam
B. Alprazolam
C. Diazepam
D. Oxazepam
E. Triazolam

104. Which of the following depot antipsychotic drugs is not prepared as an ester (decanoate)?

A. Flupenthixol
B. Fluspirilene
C. Fluphenazine
D. Clopenthixol
E. Haloperidol

105. Which one of the following antidepressant medications requires the longest washout period before switching a patient to a monoamine oxidase inhibitor antidepressant?

A. Citalopram
B. Paroxetine
C. Sertraline
D. Fluoxetine
E. Escitalopram

101. Answer: E.

Chlormethiazole has an elimination half-life ($t_{1/2}$) of less than one hour. The $t_{1/2}$ of tranylcypromine is less than two hours. Trazodone and lithium's half-lives are 4 and 13 hours respectively. Haloperidol's elimination half-life is between 12 and 38 hours. (1, pp 141–7)

102. Answer: B.

Fluoxetine has non-linear pharmacodynamic properties. This means that higher doses may produce much greater increases in plasma drug concentrations than would otherwise be expected, making titration difficult. In contract, citalopram, escitalopram, sertraline and amfebutamone (bupropion) show linear and dose-proportional pharmacokinetics, so that plasma concentrations of these drugs are proportional to the daily dose administered and are, therefore, predictable. (2) (3, pp 307–30)

103. Answer: E.

Triazolam has the shortest elimination half-life (3–5 hours) of the benzodiazepines listed. The half-lives for diazepam, lorazepam, alprazolam and oxazepam are 50–150, 10–18, 12–15 and 4–10 hours respectively. (4, pp 364–82)

104. Answer: B.

Fluspirilene is a diphenylbutylpiperidine with a long half-life and is administered as a particle suspension. In contrast, flupenthixol, fluphenazine, clopenthixol and haloperidol are all prepared as ester decanoates. (5, p 390)

105. Answer: D.

Fluoxetine requires a washout period of 5-6 weeks when switching a patient from fluoxetine to a monoamine oxidase inhibitor antidepressant, while sertraline and paroxetine each require two weeks, and citalopram and escitalopram each require one week. (6, pp 235–6)

106. Which one of the following antidepressant drugs has the least number of active metabolites?

A. Citalopram
B. Fluoxetine
C. Sertraline
D. Amitriptyline
E. Mirtazapine

107. Which one of the following psychotropic medications is least affected by haemodialysis?

A. Venlafaxine
B. Lithium
C. Sodium valproate
D. Alprazolam
E. Sertraline

108. Which of the following types of antidepressant medications is most strongly associated with anti-adrenergic side effects?

A. Selective serotonin reuptake inhibitors
B. Tetracyclic antidepressants
C. Tricyclic antidepressants
D. Monoamine oxidase inhibitors
E. St. John's wort

109. Ninety per cent of cases of medication-induced parkinsonism become apparent within which one of the following time periods?

A. Three days
B. One week
C. Three months
D. Six months
E. One year

110. Which of the following drugs is the least likely to cause drug-induced dystonic reactions in adults?

A. Fluphenazine
B. Metoclopramide
C. Olanzapine
D. Amoxapine
E. Chlorphenamine

111. Which one of the following drug classes has been least associated with an increased risk of falling in the elderly?

A. Sedatives
B. Antidepressants
C. Benzodiazepines
D. Hypnotics
E. Antihypertensives

106. Answer: C. Sertraline has no known active metabolites. Citalopram and amitriptyline have several active metabolites, including desmethylcitalopram and nortriptyline respectively; fluoxetine metabolises to norfluoxetine and mirtazapine metabolises to desmethylmirtazapine. (7)

107. Answer: A. Venlafaxine is not removed by haemodialysis. Lithium undergoes considerable removal by haemodialysis; valproate acid undergoes modest removal and both alprazolam and sertraline undergo minimal removal by haemodialysis. (7)

108. Answer: D. Monoamine oxidase inhibitors are antidepressants most strongly associated with anti-adrenergic side effects such as dry mouth, bradycardia, dizziness and drowsiness. The tricyclic antidepressant class of medications are the next most likely. Tetracyclic antidepressants (e.g., mianserin) may cause some anti-adrenergic effects. SSRIs and St. John's wort are not considered to be associated with anti-adrenergic side effects. (1, p 162, 8)

109. Answer: C. Ninety per cent of cases of medication-induced parkinsonism become apparent within the first 10 weeks of treatment. (9, p 77)

110. Answer: E. Chlorphenamine is an anti-histamine and has not been reported to cause dystonic reactions in adults. Dystonic reactions are caused by drugs that have dopamine receptor-blocking properties. Fluphenazine, metoclopramide, olanzapine and amoxapine have all got variable dopamine receptor affinity and have been associated with causing dystonic reactions in adults. (10)

111. Answer: E. A recent review examined the effects of prescribed medication on risk of falling in the elderly and generally concurred with the results of previous meta-analyses on this subject. Antihypertensives are the least likely to be associated with an increased risk of falling but in order of reducing effect, antidepressants, benzodiazepines, sedatives and hypnotics are all variably associated with significantly increased risk. (11, pp 1952–60)

112. Weight gain is most likely to occur in which one of the following antidepressants?

A. Paroxetine
B. Fluoxetine
C. Venlafaxine
D. Sertraline
E. Amfebutamone (bupropion)

113. Which one of the following cranial nerves is least likely to exit from the superior orbital fissure?

A. Oculomotor nerve
B. Abducens nerve
C. Trochlear nerve
D. Ophthalmic (first) branch of the trigeminal nerve
E. Facial nerve

114. Which one of the following cranial nerves is least likely to receive sensory input from the spinal trigeminal nucleus?

A. V
B. VII
C. VIII
D. IX
E. X

115. Which one of the following tracts is least likely to be involved in the extrapyramidal pathway?

A. Tectospinal
B. Corticospinal
C. Reticulospinal
D. Vestibulospinal
E. Rubrospinal

116. Which of the following clinical features best indicates a dominant (usually left)-sided parietal lobe lesion?

A. Ocular apraxia
B. Tactile agnosia
C. Anosognosia
D. Optic ataxia
E. Agraphia

117. Which one of the following genetic conditions is least likely to result from autosomal abnormalities?

A. Edwards' syndrome
B. Down's syndrome
C. Turner syndrome
D. Patau's syndrome
E. Cri-du-chat syndrome

112. Answer: A. Paroxetine has been consistently reported to be the SSRI most associated with increased weight gain. Venlafaxine has been generally reported to have little or no effect on weight gain and bupropion treatment has been associated with weight loss. (6, pp 235–6, 12, pp 15–25)

113. Answer: E. The facial nerve exits from the internal auditory meatus. The oculomotor, abducens, trochlear and trigeminal (ophthalmic branch) nerves all exit the skull from the superior orbital fissure. (13, p 22)

114. Answer: C. The spinal trigeminal nucleus is involved in subserving sensory functions for the V (trigeminal–opthalmic branch), VII (facial), IX (glossopharyngeal) and X (vagus) cranial nerves. (13, p 24)

115. Answer: B. The corticospinal tract provides excitatory input to anterior horn cells of the spinal cord. In contrast the extrapyramidal pathway tract system (tectospinal, reticulospinal, vestibulospinal and rubrospinal) are tracts that pass motor impulses from the cerebral cortex to the spinal cord and tend to be inhibitory. (1, p 43)

116. Answer: E. Lesions in the dominant (usually left) parietal lobe can result in Gerstmann's syndrome, which includes right-left confusion, difficulty with writing (agraphia) and difficulty with mathematics (acalculia). It also can lead to tactile agnosia and conduction aphasia while non-dominant (usually right)-sided parietal lobe lesions can result in contralateral neglect, tactile agnosia, anosodiaphoria and anosognosia. Bilateral lesions can lead to Balint's syndrome, a visual attention and motor syndrome that includes ocular apraxia, optic ataxia and simultanagnosia. (14, p 110, 15)

117. Answer: C. Turner syndrome results from a sex chromosome abnormality (genotype: 45, XO). In contrast, Edwards' syndrome (trisomy 18), Down's syndrome (trisomy 21), Patau's syndrome (trisomy 13) and Cri-du-chat syndrome (partial deletion of the short arm of chromosome 5) are autosomal abnormalities. (14, pp 188–9)

118. Which one of the following disorders is least likely inherited in an autosomal recessive manner?

    A. Friedrich's ataxia
    B. Wilson's disease
    C. Galactosaemia
    D. Neurofibromatosis
    E. Niemann–Pick disease

119. Which one of the following statements is most true?

    A. Obsessive compulsive disorder has a heritability of 85%.
    B. Gilles de la Tourette's syndrome has been associated with linkage to 15q21.
    C. Angelman's syndrome involves a 'parent-of-origin' effect.
    D. In ADHD, males are affected four times more than females.
    E. Twin studies of dyslexia show that deficits in reading have a higher heritability than spelling deficits.

120. Which one of the following statements relating to premenstrual syndrome (PMS) is least correct?

    A. Up to 40% of women experience some premenstrual symptoms.
    B. Twenty per cent of women experiencing PMS report that the symptoms impact on their lives.
    C. PMS does not occur after oophorectomy.
    D. Psychosocial factors are believed not to be the primary cause.
    E. Prevalence is positively associated with increased parity.

121. Which of the following statements relating to disorders of pregnancy is least correct?

    A. Couvade syndrome has been described in the male partner of the pregnant female.
    B. In the general population, 10% of women become depressed in the first few months after delivery of their baby.
    C. Clomipramine can be especially helpful in the treatment of post-natal depression with associated panic disorder.
    D. The progesterone deficiency hypothesis is associated with both 'baby blues' and post-natal depression.
    E. Puerperal psychosis commonly starts within 48 hours of delivery.

122. Which of the following statements is least true?

    A. Twenty to forty per cent of seasonal affective disorder sufferers report a positive family history of affective disorder.
    B. Ten per cent of those who initially suffer a depressive episode subsequently develop mania.
    C. Falret described 'folie circulaire' in relation to bipolar affective disorder.
    D. 'Bell's mania' describes cases of mania where there is rapid onset of confusional symptoms without obvious evidence of underlying physical illness.
    E. Five to ten per cent of bipolar affective disorder is accounted for by unipolar mania.

118. Answer: D. Neurofibromatosis is an autosomal dominant disorder. In contrast, Niemann–Pick disease, Friedrich's ataxia, Wilson's disease and galactosaemia are inherited in an autosomal recessive manner. (14, pp 189–91)

119. Answer: C. Angelman's syndrome involves a parent-of-origin effect also known as imprinting. Obsessive compulsive disorder has a heritability of approximately 70%. Gilles de la Tourette's syndrome has been associated with linkage to 11q23. In ADHD, males are affected three times more than females. Twin studies of dyslexia show that deficits in spelling have a higher heritability than reading deficits. (13, pp 62–3)

120. Answer: B. All of the statements provided are correct with the exception of B. Five to ten per cent of women experiencing PMS report significant or severe symptoms that impact adversely on their lives. (5, p 942, 14, pp 302–4)

121. Answer: E. The statements provided are correct with the exception of E. Puerperal psychosis usually starts within four to five days post partum with development of symptoms such as confusion and affective changes. (5, pp 904, 920–7, 14, pp 297, 302–4, 307–10)

122. Answer: A. All statements provided are correct with the exception of A. More than 50% of those suffering from seasonal affective disorder report a positive family history of affective disorder. (5, pp 33, 42, 51, 56, 58)

123. In relation to psychological theory, which one of the following statements is least true?

    A.   Rationalisation is said to occur in psychotic states.

    B.   According to Freud, primary process thinking is rational and follows principles of logic, time and space.

    C.   Ego defence mechanisms are unconscious and sometimes pathological.

    D.   Turning against oneself is an example of a displacement defence mechanism.

    E.   The defence mechanism of projective identification has been associated with paranoid mental states.

124. Which one of the following statements relating to psychoanalytic thought is least correct?

    A.   Melanie Klein initially described the notion of 'projective identification'.

    B.   Alfred Adler argued that neurosis originated in trying to cope with feelings of inferiority.

    C.   Wilfred Bion described 'basic assumptions' generated automatically in groups of people.

    D.   Jacques Lacan described a developmental stage which he called the 'symbolic order'.

    E.   Margaret Mahler described the 'false self'.

125. According to findings of the CATIE trial comparing antipsychotic treatments in the treatment of schizophrenia, which of the following statements is least true?

    A.   Olanzapine was found to be significantly more effective than risperidone.

    B.   Olanzapine was associated with the most adverse metabolic effects.

    C.   Perphenazine was found to be as clinically effective as the other antipsychotics and the most cost-effective drug.

    D.   There were obvious differences in risk of developing tardive dyskinesia across treatment groups.

    E.   Ziprasidone had the least propensity to weight gain.

126. Regarding treatment of unipolar depressive disorder in adults, which one of the following statements is least true?

    A.   Approximately two-thirds of patients with depressive disorder are treated successfully with antidepressant medication alone.

    B.   Combined treatment with antidepressant medication and cognitive behavioural therapy (CBT) confers an additional treatment effect of approximately 30% over treatment with each treatment alone.

    C.   Relapse rates following treatment discontinuation are higher in those taking medication compared with those who have received CBT.

    D.   CBT is just as effective in the treatment of severe depressive disorder as antidepressant medication.

    E.   Interpersonal therapy and CBT have been found to be equally effective in the treatment of major depressive disorder.

123. Answer: B. The statements provided are correct with the exception of B. Freud posited that there were two principles of mental functioning – primary and secondary processes – and that of these, primary process thinking occurs in infantile life, dreaming and fantasy. (13, pp 250–5, 14, p 103)

124. Answer: E. The statements provided are correct with the exception of E. Donald Winnicott described the concept of the 'false self' in terms in mother-baby separation. (13, pp 257–61)

125. Answer: D. The statements provided are correct with the exception of D. There were no significant differences between the selected antipsychotic medications evaluated in the CATIE trial in terms of relative risk to developing tardive dyskinesia. (16)

126. Answer: D. The statements provided are correct with the exception of D. CBT has been found to be slightly less effective than antidepressant therapy in the treatment of unipolar major depressive disorder and is recommended as equally efficacious in the treatment of mild-to-moderate unipolar depressive disorder. (17)

127. A 35-year-old man was admitted with severe depressive symptoms and psychosis. Medications on admission were venlafaxine slow release 225 mg daily. Olanzapine 10 mg and mirtazapine 15 mg were added. He became anxious, tremulous and confused. Examination revealed a tachycardia, excessive sweating, hypertension, pyrexia hyperreflexia, rigidity and clonus in the lower limbs. There was raised CK-MM. Which is the best fit diagnosis?

A. Malignant catatonia
B. Malignant hyperpyrexia
C. Neuroleptic malignant syndrome
D. Sepsis
E. Serotonin syndrome

128. A 50-year-old woman is referred by her GP with her second episode of depressive illness. She is otherwise healthy, but she has a history of hyponatraemia on sertraline in the past. In view of her history, which antidepressant would you consider the safest choice?

A. Duloxetine
B. Escitalopram
C. Fluoxetine
D. Mirtazapine
E. Moclobemide

129. Which of the following characteristics would be least likely to assist in diagnosing DSM IV criteria for paranoid personality disorder?

A. Is reluctant to confide in others.
B. Odd thinking and speech.
C. Persistently bearing grudges.
D. Reads hidden or threatening meanings into benign remarks.
E. Suspects without sufficient basis that others are exploiting them.

130. In considering the current available evidence for risk factors for the condition known as postpartum psychosis, which of the following is least likely to be associated with its development?

A. Experiencing an obstetric complication during delivery.
B. First-degree relative who has experienced an episode of puerperal psychosis.
C. History of bipolar disorder.
D. Primiparity.
E. Psychosocial stressors.

131. A 26-year-old woman with a history of schizophrenia presents with a relapse of psychosis, due to non-compliance with medication. She has a history of hepatitis C infection and liver function tests are abnormal with moderate impairment. All other routine blood tests are normal. She is on no medication. Which of the following antipsychotic medications would be the most suitable to treat her symptoms?

A. Amisulpride
B. Chlorpromazine
C. Flupenthixol decanoate
D. Quetiapine
E. Risperidone

127. Answer: E.   Hyperreflexia and clonus, particularly in the lower extremities, are more likely to occur in serotonin syndrome than in the other conditions. A raised CK can occur in all of the above diagnoses. Malignant hyperpyrexia is a condition in which genetically predisposed individuals have a hypersensitive reaction to some anaesthetics. Neuroleptic malignant syndrome and malignant catatonia are thought to have almost identical clinical features, except that there is a history of exposure to dopamine antagonists in the former. (18)

128. Answer: E.   Most antidepressants have been associated with hyponatraemia as indeed have antipsychotics and carbamazepine. MAOIs, however, appear to have a lower number of reports associating them with hyponatreamia. The Maudsley Guidelines suggest a trial of a noradrenergic drug or an MAOI like moclobemide, with close monitoring of serum sodium. (6, pp 210–1)

129. Answer: B.   Both schizotypal personality disorder and paranoid personality disorder have traits of suspiciousness and interpersonal coldness/aloofness in common. However, 'odd thinking and speech' is a criterion for schizotypal personality disorder. Schizoid personality disorder also has the trait of emotional coldness, but does not usually have paranoid ideation. (19, pp 690–4)

130. Answer: E.   Stressful life events have consistently been shown not to be associated with the development of puerperal psychosis in women at high risk of same, whereas answers A–D inclusive have all been found to be associated with it. (20)

131. Answer: A.   Amisulpride is the drug of choice as it is predominantly renally excreted and should be safe as long as renal function is normal. Flupenthixol and quetiapine are both hepatically metabolised, and caution is recommended in hepatic impairment. Chlorpromazine is known for its propensity to cause liver toxicity and should not be administered in hepatic impairment. A maximum dose of 4 mg risperidone is recommended in hepatic impairment according to the Maudsley Guidelines. (6, pp 404–5)

132. A 63-year-old right-handed man was referred to the local CMHT for assessment. Collateral history reported that the man, who previously had been a keen artist, now seemed to paint only on the right side of the canvas. He was no longer able to set the table or put on his clothes properly. His memory seemed intact. Neuroimaging was requested and revealed a malignant brain tumour. Based on the information above, which of the following areas of the brain are the most likely sites for the tumour?

    A.   Diencephalon and brainstem
    B.   Dominant parietal lobe
    C.   Dominant temporal lobe
    D.   Non-dominant parietal lobe
    E.   Orbitofrontal area

133. This drug acts as a potent antagonist at the $alpha_1$ and H_1 receptors and to a moderate degree at the $5HT_{2A}$, D_2 receptors and the muscarinic cholinergic receptors. It has a low affinity for the nigrostriatal dopaminergic neurons. It does not elevate serum prolactin. Which of the following drugs most closely matches the above profile?

    A.   Amisulpride
    B.   Aripiprazole
    C.   Clozapine
    D.   Quetiapine
    E.   Risperidone

134. On considering the distribution of dementias among those under the age of 65 years compared with those over that age, which dementia in particular occurs more commonly as an early onset dementia than a late onset one?

    A.   Alzheimer's dementia
    B.   Dementia with Lewy bodies
    C.   Fronto-temporal dementia
    D.   Mixed dementia
    E.   Vascular dementia

135. A 70-year-old woman is referred to the CMHT for evaluation of a one-year history of progressive cognitive decline. The woman's husband says that her cognition appears to fluctuate; at times her concentration and attention appear quite good but at other times appear very poor. According to McKeith, which of the following features if also present would most strongly support the diagnosis of dementia with Lewy bodies (DLB)?

    A.   Evidence of stroke from focal neurological signs or brain imaging
    B.   Neuroleptic sensitivity
    C.   Repeated falls
    D.   Spontaneous motor features of parkinsonism
    E.   Transient loss of consciousness

132. Answer: D.

In the example above the patient neglects the contralateral half of space. He has dressing dyspraxia and there is evidence of visuospatial disorganisation, all typical of non-dominant parietal lobe lesions. Lesions of the dominant parietal lobe produce deficits in keeping with Gerstmann's syndrome. Dominant temporal lobe lesions may produce a sensory aphasia, while lesions of the orbitofrontal area may produce symptoms of irritability, impulsivity and antisocial behaviour. Lesions of the deep midline structures usually present with an amnestic syndrome and hypersomnia. (21, pp 492–4)

133. Answer: D.

Clozapine, though structurally similar to quetiapine, has only a weak affinity for D_2 but binds more strongly to D_4 and has a strong affinity for serotonergic receptors such as $5HT_{2A}$ and $5HT_{2C}$. Amisulpride is a pure D_2 and D_3 antagonist. Aripiprazole is a partial agonist at D_2 and $5HT_{1A}$ receptors. Risperidone has potent $5HT_2$ antagonistic action, with a high affinity for D_2 receptors. As the dosage increases, it can cause extrapyramidal side effects and high prolactin levels. (21, pp 248–50)

134. Answer: C.

Fronto-temporal dementia accounts for approximately 13% of dementias in the under 65 year age group compared to 2% of the over 65 year age group. Alzheimer's disease is the most common dementia type in both age groups, accounting for 31% in the younger age group and 62% in the older age group. Vascular dementia is the second most common dementia in the under 65 year age group and also in the over 65 year age group. DLB comprises about 4% of the dementias in both age groups. (22)

135. Answer: D.

According to the Consensus criteria for the clinical diagnosis of probable and possible dementia with Lewy bodies, answers B, C and E are all features suggestive of the diagnosis, but answer D is one of the three core features, two of which are required for a probable diagnosis of DLB. Answer A is incorrect; if present it is more suggestive of a vascular dementia. (21, p 515)

136. A 30-year-old woman was referred to a psychotherapist for treatment of depression. The initial assessment revealed that a key focus for this lady was grief, as her father had died suddenly six months earlier. The therapist ascertained that she would benefit from a structured time-limited therapy, using a collaborative approach. Emphasis would be on the here and now. However, the client felt that she would be unable to engage in regular, formal 'homework'. Which of the following psychotherapies would be the most suitable for this client, considering the above information?

A. Cognitive analytic therapy
B. Cognitive behavioural therapy
C. Interpersonal therapy
D. Psychoanalytic psychotherapy
E. Supportive psychotherapy

137. In considering the disorder 'pathological fire-setting' in ICD-10, which of the following statements is least true?

A. An intense interest in watching fires burn may be present.
B. Feeling of increasing tension before the act and excitement after the act may occur.
C. Fires are typically started in response to delusional ideas and command hallucinations.
D. Repeated fire-setting occurs without any obvious motive.
E. There may be an abnormal interest in fire engines.

138. In considering obsessive compulsive disorder, which of the following statements is least true?

A. A bimodal age of onset with peaks occurs at ages 12–14 years and 20–22 years.
B. Brain imaging shows morphological changes in basal ganglia structure.
C. First-degree relatives have a higher than normal incidence of psychiatric disorders.
D. Predominance of phobic ruminative ideas and absence of compulsions is a poor prognostic factor.
E. Relapse often follows discontinuation of pharmacological treatment.

139. On considering the results of Kendall's study (1987) on the epidemiology of puerperal psychosis, which of the following statements is least correct?

A. An association with caesarean birth was identified.
B. If considering primagravid women only, the relative risk of hospital admission increased to 35 in the first month after delivery.
C. Rate of puerperal psychosis was 4.8 per 1000 deliveries.
D. The relative rate of hospital admission decreased in pregnancy 0.65.
E. The relative risk of hospital admission was 22 in the first month after delivery.

136. Answer: C.

Interpersonal therapy satisfies all the above criteria for the required form of therapy. IPT does not involve homework per se as in CBT, but patients are encouraged to try out new skills or develop their social network in between sessions. Note that apart from this woman not wishing to engage in homework, the second closest correct answer would have been B (CBT). Both therapies A and C involve references to past experiences, and collaborative psycho therapy E is less structured and collaborative. (23)

137. Answer: C.

Features A, B and D must all be present before a diagnosis of pathological fire-setting can be made. This disorder is sometimes accompanied by the individual having an abnormal interest in fire engines and the associated firefighting equipment. The diagnosis of pathological fire-setting cannot be made if the fire-setting occurs in the context of schizophrenia. (24, p 212)

138. Answer: D.

This is in fact a favourable prognostic factor. Answers A, B, C and E are all true. (14, p 291)

139. Answer: C.

The rate of puerperal psychosis identified by Kendal's study was 1 per 1000 deliveries. Janssen's study in Sweden (1964) reported a rate of 4.8 per 1000 admissions to a university hospital (Answer C). It is thought that a greater availability of hospital beds and a lower threshold for admission may account for the different rates. All the other answers are correct. (21, p 637)

140. The replication study of the National Comorbidity Survey in the U.S. by Kessler (2005) and the study by Wittchen and Jacobi (2005), which looked at the frequency and burden of mental disorders in Europe, produced a number of interesting results. Which one of the following results is least true?

    A. Lifetime prevalence for social phobia in the U.S. study was almost twice that reported in the European study.

    B. Median age of onset for specific phobias was 7 years according to the U.S. study.

    C. Median age of onset for substance abuse was 20 years according to the U.S. study.

    D. Panic disorder was equally prevalent among the sexes across all the age bands in the European study.

    E. The lifetime prevalence of post-traumatic stress disorder was estimated to be 6.8% according to the U.S. study.

141. On considering the neuroanatomy of the spinal cord, which of the following statements is least correct?

    A. Discriminative touch and proprioception are carried in the ipsilateral posterior white column.

    B. Light touch and pressure sensations are carried in the ipsilateral anterior spinothalamic tract.

    C. Pain and temperature sensations are carried in the contralateral lateral spinothalamic tracts.

    D. The average spinal cord is approximately 45 cm long.

    E. Thirty-one pairs of spinal nerves are attached to the spinal cord.

142. Regarding amino acids that have been found to act as central neurotransmitters, which of the following statements is least correct?

    A. GABA is an inhibitory amino acids that causes hyperpolarisation of neurons.

    B. The excitatory amino acids include glutamic acid and glycine.

    C. GABA has been found to be reduced in the brain cell of Huntington's disease.

    D. NMDA is an agonist of some glutamic acid receptors.

    E. NMDA antagonists may be clinically useful in Alzheimer's disease.

143. A young man with epilepsy is admitted into an epilepsy monitoring unit for continuous EEG and video monitoring because his seizure frequency has increased. Which of the following is the least commonly used EEG-activating procedure used to expose EEG abnormalities?

    A. Hyperventilation for 2–3 minutes

    B. Photic stimulation

    C. Use of drugs to induce sleep

    D. Sleep deprivation

    E. Valsalva manoeuvre

140. Answer: D.

Panic disorder is 3.4 times more common in women than in men below the age of 34, but the prevalence becomes approximately equal after the age of 50 years, according to the study by Wittchen and Jacobi (2005). However, this study showed that agoraphobia (without panic), social phobia and specific phobia were more common in women than men across all age bands. All the other statements are correct. Of note, a lifetime prevalence for PTSD could not be calculated in the European study. (21, p 319)

141. Answer: B.

The anterior spinothalamic tract conveys light touch and pressure sense, while the lateral spinothalamic tracts are concerned with transmission of pain and temperature. After entering the posterior roots and before entering the anterior and lateral spinothalamic tracts, the sensory fibres ascend a short distance before crossing over to ascend in the contralateral tracts. However, the fibres carrying discriminative touch, proprioception and vibration sensation pass mainly uncrossed to the cuneate and gracile nuclei in the medulla oblongata. The other statements are all correct. (1, pp 4–5)

142. Answer: B.

The excitatory amino acids that cause depolarisation of neurons include glutamic acid, aspartic acid, cysteic acid and homocysteic acid. The inhibitory amino acids include GABA and glycine, and they cause hyperpolarisation in neurones. NMDA (*N*-methyl-d-aspartic acid) receptors are a form of glutamic acid receptors. Memantine is an NMDA receptor antagonist used in the management of moderate to severe Alzheimer's dementia. GABA has been found to be reduced in the brains of patients with Huntington's disease and Alzheimer's disease. (1, pp 117–8)

143. Answer: E.

EEG-activating procedures are used to demonstrate EEG abnormalities that are either not obvious on a normal EEG reading or present but not clear. Hyperventilation for 2–3 minutes is believed to cause cerebral hypoxia, which leads to cortical hyperexcitability, which in turn may cause high-amplitude delta activity in patients with epilepsy. A stroboscope may be used to produce light flashes of a variable frequency, which can induce seizure activity in those at risk. A patient, who is partially sleep-deprived, is more likely to fall asleep during the EEG recording and seizure activity can then occur. Drugs like pentobarbitone can also be used to induce sleep and thus allow seizure activity to emerge as the patient passes through the different stages of sleep. The Valsalva manoeuvre is not routinely used to induce seizures. However, it can cause dizziness and syncope in some individuals. (1, p 84)

144. Which of the following statements regarding EEG rhythms is least true?

    A. When an adult human is awake but the eyes are closed, the normal resting EEG rhythm is composed of alpha activity.

    B. Delta activity has a frequency of less than 4 hertz per second.

    C. During loss of consciousness from a general anaesthetic, theta activity is prominent.

    D. High-frequency beta activity is present when an individual is very alert.

    E. EEG recordings from newborn infants may be recognised by the relative lack of electrical activity.

145. Regarding genetically inherited disorders, which of the following pairings are least correct?

    A. Acute intermittent porphyria and autosomal dominance inheritance.

    B. Fragile X syndrome and X-linked dominant inheritance.

    C. Huntington's chorea and autosomal dominance inheritance.

    D. Phenylketonuria and autosomal recessive inheritance.

    E. Wilson's disease and autosomal recessive inheritance.

146. Regarding the macroscopic findings of the following conditions, which of the following pairings is least correct?

    A. Alzheimer's disease with global atrophy of the brain and widened sulci and ventricular enlargement.

    B. Huntington's chorea and marked atrophy of the corpus striatum, basal ganglia and the caudate nucleus.

    C. Pick disease and selective asymmetrical atrophy of the frontal and temporal lobes.

    D. Wernicke's encephalopathy and lesions in the mammillary bodies.

    E. Wilson's disease and depigmentation of the substantia nigra, particularly of the zona compacta.

147. A 60-year-old man presents with severe stabbing pains in his legs lasting a few seconds. He walks with a wide-based and stomping gait. On neurological examination, there is absence of proprioception and vibration sensation in the lower limbs. Assuming the diagnosis is tabes dorsalis, which of the following clinical or pathological findings are least likely to be found in this patient?

    A. Argyll Robertson pupil

    B. Charcot's joint

    C. Frontal lobe personality changes

    D. Granulomatous lesions may be attached to the meninges and the underlying part of the brain.

    E. Histologically, the cerebral cortex has a spongy appearance and is identified by the presence of multiple vacuoles.

148. Regarding the epidemiology of somatisation disorder, which of the following statements is least correct?

    A. A history of parents with frequent complaints of poor physical health has been identified.

    B. A history of physical and sexual abuse has been found in patients with this condition.

    C. Bass and May (2002) claimed that 4% of the general population and 9% of those admitted into tertiary care have a history of multiple chronic functional somatic symptoms.

    D. It has not been found to be associated with a history of unexplained symptoms in childhood.

    E. It is twice as common in women.

144. Answer: C.

Delta activity is typical during loss of consciousness caused by a general anaesthetic. When an adult human is awake with closed eyes, alpha activity is prominent. On opening the eyes and becoming more alert, this is replaced by beta activity. When a person becomes drowsy and is in light sleep, theta activity occurs. In deep sleep, delta activity is more prominent. Of note, normal EEG rhythms vary with age. As a child gets older, the waking delta and theta activities are gradually replaced by the adult alpha rhythm. (1, pp 82–4)

145. Answer: B.

Fragile X syndrome is an X-linked recessive disorder. In this condition, male-to-male transmission generally does not occur and female heterozygotes are carriers. Acute intermittent porphyria and Huntington's chorea are both inherited in an autosomal dominant manner. Phenylketonuria is an autosomal recessive disorder of protein metabolism, and Wilson's disease, also known as hepatolenticular degeneration, is also inherited this way. (1, pp 178–84)

146. Answer: E.

Wilson's disease is an autosomal recessive disorder of copper metabolism. It is characterised pathologically by brownish discolouration (due to copper deposition) and atrophy in the basal ganglia. In Parkinson's disease the macroscopic findings are depigmentation of the substantia nigra. All the other statements and pairings are correct. (1, pp 223–8)

147. Answer: E.

These cerebral cortex findings are found more specifically in Creutzfeldt–Jakob disease. Argyll Robertson pupils is a condition where the pupils are small and irregular, there is no light reflex, but the pupils do constrict with accommodation. It is due to a syphilitic lesion and an interruption of the fibres from the pretectal nucleus to the Edinger–Westphal nucleus. Tabes dorsalis can also occur in neurosyphilis; there may be a loss of deep pain sensation that can lead to neuropathic joints. Frontal lobe personality changes can occur in General Paralysis of the Insane and the granulomatous lesions are typical of the syphilitic gummas that can occur in the cerebral hemispheres or cerebellum. (1, pp 212–4)

148. Answer: D.

In fact an association has been found between a history of unexplained physical symptoms in childhood and an adult diagnosis of somatisation disorder. A community prevalence rate of 0.4% was found in 1986 (Swartz et al.), where strict criteria for somatisation disorder were used. A subsequent primary care study reported a prevalence rate of 1–2%. However when less strict criteria were used, a smaller number of symptoms were required to make the diagnosis and the prevalence rate increased as seen in Bass and May's study. All of the other statements are correct. (21, pp 397–8)

149. A 30-year-old man presents with his second psychotic episode, the first occurring a year earlier. Collateral history reveals that he has a history of epilepsy. Which of the following facts would most support a diagnosis of schizophrenia?

    A. He first developed seizures when he was 15 years old.
    B. His affect on examination is blunted.
    C. His premorbid personality remains intact.
    D. There is an increased incidence of neurological abnormality on examination.
    E. There is no increased family history of schizophrenia.

150. Regarding the psychiatric aspects of epilepsy, which of the following statements is least correct?

    A. Approximately 20% of patients with 'intractable epilepsy' have non-epileptic seizures, though these may coexist with true epilepsy.
    B. Depression and anxiety are the most common interictal psychiatric disorders.
    C. Elation is the most common ictal emotion.
    D. SSRIs may cause an increase in the level of phenytoin and carbamazepine.
    E. The suicide risk is increased fivefold in those with epilepsy.

151. Regarding long-acting depot preparations, which of the following statements is least correct?

    A. Flupenthixol decanoate has a wide therapeutic dose range.
    B. Fluphenazine is the only depot drug that produces an abrupt but transient rise in drug levels after injection.
    C. Haloperidol decanoate has a half-life of about three weeks.
    D. Maximum dosage for zuclopenthixol decanoate is 600 mg weekly.
    E. Pipotiazine palmitate produces more extrapyramidal side effects than fluphenazine.

152. Which of the following statements is most true with regard to motivational interviewing?

    A. Was pioneered by Abraham Maslow.
    B. Works with the assumption that patients often display defence mechanisms.
    C. Is confrontational in style.
    D. Attempts to develop discrepancy in the client.
    E. Has been shown to be of little use in the contemplation phase of change.

149. Answer: B.

Chronic interictal psychosis may often resemble schizophrenia in its clinical presentation. The typical picture is one of a paranoid psychosis associated with hallucinations and often there is evidence of first-rank symptoms. There are, however, a number of features that help differentiate it from schizophrenia. Generally the psychosis develops some 10–15 years after the development of epilepsy. The premorbid personality remains intact and the affect is usually warm. There is often an increased incidence of neurological abnormality on examination and there is usually no family history of schizophrenia. (21, pp 528–9)

150. Answer: C.

The most common ictal emotion is actually fear. If not remembered by the patient, witnesses usually recall that the patient often looked terrified during the seizure. Depression is also a common ictal emotion whereas elation is rare. Non-epileptic attack disorders often coexist in patients with real epilepsy and in fact patients with epilepsy are one of the groups most likely to have them. It has been estimated that the lifetime prevalence of depression is about 62% in those with epilepsy, compared with 17% in the general population. One study also suggested that the suicide risk is increased by a factor of five. SSRIs are commonly used in the treatment of depression in epilepsy, and though the interactions mentioned above are theoretically possible, they are rarely of clinical significance. (21, pp 528–30)

151. Answer: E.

It produces less extrapyramidal side effects than fluphenazine. The maximum licensed dose of flupenthixol is 400 mg per week, according to the BNF, which is actually 20 times higher than the commonly administered dose of 40 mg per fortnight. Fluphenazine decanoate can cause acute dystonic reactions within the first 24 hours following the injection, as a consequence of the abrupt rise in blood levels of the drug. Haloperidol decanoate can be given every 6–8 weeks in some patients because of its long half-life. The maximum dose of zuclopenthixol decanoate is 600 mg weekly. (21, pp 250–2)

152. Answer: D.

Motivational interviewing assumes that many clients are still ambivalent about their motivation to change when they consult for treatment. The technique therefore uses the key principles of expressing empathy, developing discrepancy, rolling with resistance, and supporting self-efficacy to enhance intrinsic motivation to change by exploring and resolving ambivalence. It tries to avoid a defensive reaction of patients to advice or instruction. The interview model is described as 'confrontational in purpose but not in style'. The technique was pioneered by Miller and is most useful in the pre-contemplation and contemplation stages of change. Abraham Maslow developed a hierarchy of needs to explain human motivation (A). Defence mechanisms are concepts used in psychodynamic psychotherapy (B). (25, pp 126–7)

153. Which of the following statements is most true relating to women performing better than men on IQ tests?

   A.   In fewer IQ subtests than two decades ago.
   B.   In IQ subtests requiring mathematical skills.
   C.   In total IQ scores.
   D.   In IQ subtests requiring visuospatial skills.
   E.   In IQ subtests requiring motor skills involving aiming.

154. In learning theory, the term *contingency* best refers to which of the following?

   A.   The relationship between an event and an emotional response.
   B.   The relationship between the behaviour and its consequence.
   C.   An event that increases the probability of a response when presented after it.
   D.   A form of learning in which a voluntary response is increased or decreased, depending on positive and negative consequences.
   E.   Responses that work on the environment to change it.

155. Which of the following statements is most true regarding mirtazapine?

   A.   Activates central H_1 histamine receptors.
   B.   Has high affinity to muscarinic cholinoceptors.
   C.   Has little affinity to central α_2-adrenoceptors.
   D.   Blocks $5\text{-}HT_2$ and $5\text{-}HT_3$ receptors.
   E.   Selectively enhances the release of serotonin.

156. In neurons, lithium has been shown to be least likely to modulate which of the following systems?

   A.   Noradrenaline-induced cAMP activity.
   B.   Neuroleptic-induced hypersensitivity of dopamine receptors.
   C.   The phosphoinositol (PI) second messenger system.
   D.   The protein C kinase (PKC) signalling system.
   E.   Muscarinic cholinoceptor activation.

157. When euthymic volunteers are given tricyclic antidepressant (TCA) medications, which of the following statements is most true?

   A.   The medication causes transient elevation of mood.
   B.   The medication increases general CNS arousal.
   C.   The medication decreases total time spent in REM sleep.
   D.   The medication improves psychomotor performance.
   E.   The medication decreases the latency to the onset of REM sleep.

158. Benzodiazepine withdrawal is least associated with which of the following?

   A.   A sensation of abnormal body sway
   B.   Hyperacusis
   C.   Hypersensitivity to touch and pain
   D.   Occurrence of epileptic seizures in 15–20% of cases
   E.   Muscle twitching

153. Answer: A.

Total IQ scores for men and women show no significant statistical differences. Males perform typically better on visuospatial tasks, mathematical tasks, and motor tasks, whereas women traditionally excel in verbal abilities, fine motor tasks, and perceptual thresholds (touch, taste, hearing, olfaction). However, verbal test scores for men have converged over the last decades towards those of women, and similarly women now match the mathematical abilities of males. The only persisting gender difference remaining today is the better performance of men in visuospatial tasks. (25, p 47)

154. Answer: B.

This relationship reflects contingency, for example there is a contingency between lever-pressing and the delivery of food. Answer C is the definition of a reinforcer. Answer D is operant conditioning. The last answer applies to an operant. (25, pp 11–16)

155. Answer: D.

Mirtazapine blocks with high affinity central α_2-adrenoceptors, 5-HT$_2$ and 5-HT$_3$ receptors, and H$_1$-histamine receptors, and has little affinity for α_1-adrenoceptors and muscarinic cholinoceptors. It enhances the release of both noradrenaline and serotonin through a complex modulatory mechanism on adrenergic and serotonergic systems. H$_1$-histamine receptor-blocking is thought to cause the common side effects of drowsiness and weight gain. Rare but severe side effects include leucopenia and granulocytopenia, which can occasionally develop into agranulocytosis. (26, pp 127–8)

156. Answer: E.

The exact therapeutic mechanism of lithium is poorly understood. The drug was shown to affect brain levels of serotonin, noradrenaline and dopamine. It blocks supersensitivity of dopamine receptors, which develops after chronic inhibition by neuroleptics. On a cellular level, lithium inhibits both cAMP and PI second messenger systems. Inhibition of PI leads to activation of the protein kinase C (PKC) signalling cascade. Lithium has not been shown to modulate the cholinergic system. (26, pp 246–50)

157. Answer: C.

In non-depressed individuals, TCAs often cause sedation and dysphoria. They impair psychomotor performance and decrease CNS arousal. TCAs have profound effects on sleep. They decrease the number of awakenings, increase stage IV sleep, increase the latency to the onset of REM sleep and decrease the total time spent in REM sleep. (26, pp 202–4)

158. Answer: D.

Epileptic seizures, confusional states and hallucinations may occur in benzodiazepine withdrawal, but these are noted in less than 5% of cases. Symptoms of abnormal sensory perception, such as hyperacusis, paraesthesia, photophobia, hypersensitivity to touch and pain, occur frequently. Other somatic symptoms often include muscle stiffness or twitching. Peculiar to benzodiazepine withdrawal is a sensation of abnormal body sway. (26, pp 164–5)

159. Sodium valproate is best associated with which one of the following side effects?

    A. Weight gain
    B. Anaemia
    C. Hirsutism
    D. Nephrotoxicity
    E. Ataxia

160. Which of the following statements is most true in relation to drug development?

    A. Phase IV clinical trials are carried out when a drug is licensed but not yet marketed.
    B. Phase I clinical trials are carried out in university hospital units on a small group of very ill patients.
    C. Phase I clinical trials are carried out on healthy non-human primates.
    D. Phase II clinical trials are usually placebo controlled and double blind.
    E. In phase III, trials of usually up to 10 different doses of the drug are examined against placebos.

161. Which of the following statements is most true regarding suicide rates?

    A. Suicide rates among young adults are higher than those in the elderly.
    B. Suicide rates in the northern hemisphere are highest in autumn and winter.
    C. Suicide rates in the Western world are highest in social classes V and I.
    D. Suicide rates increased significantly in Europe during the world wars.
    E. Suicide rates among farmers are significantly lower than those in the general population.

162. Which of the following statements is most true with respect to post-mortem brains of patients with schizophrenia?

    A. Mild gliosis of the striatum is a replicated finding.
    B. Decreased numbers of oligodendroglial cells have not been found.
    C. Symmetry between the hemispheres is reduced.
    D. Synaptic structures and synaptic proteins are unaltered.
    E. Decreased numbers of hippocampal GABAergic interneurons have been reported.

159. Answer: A. Weight gain is a common side effect of sodium valproate. Other common side effects include tremor, ankle swelling, hair thinning and cognitive dysfunction. Less common side effects include hepatotoxicity and thrombocytopenia. Metabolic abnormalities such as hyperammonaemia and glycinaemia have been described. A severe but rare side effect is encephalopathy. (26, pp 269–70)

160. Answer: D. Drug development takes place in defined phases, which include the pre-clinical research and development phase (where experiments are carried out on cell cultures and animals) and the clinical phases I–IV (where experiments are carried out in humans). Phase I clinical trials are carried out on drug company premises or within a contract research organisation and include a small number of healthy volunteers to determine safety and correct dose. Phase II studies examine the drug's efficacy, and are usually carried out as placebo-controlled, double-blind trials in the patient population. In Phase III, typically one or two doses of the drug are examined in thousands of patients over prolonged periods of time to further establish efficacy and to screen for uncommon side effects. Pharma companies can then apply for licence with the relevant government authority. Phase IV trials are carried out after the drug is marketed, to extend knowledge about side effects and to possibly extend the target indications. (26, pp 78–83)

161. Answer: C. Age-wise, suicide rates of both men and women are highest in the elderly. In terms of social class, social classes V (unskilled workers) and I (professionals) have the highest rates. Certain professions such as veterinary surgeons, pharmacists and farmers have suicide rates twice as high as expected. Significantly more suicides occur in spring and early summer. During each of the world wars, suicide rates dropped throughout Europe. Being employed and being married are thought to have protective effects. (27, pp 408–10)

162. Answer: E. Neuropathological changes in schizophrenia are subtle. In contrast to many neurodegenerative disorders, there is no proliferation of astroglia (gliosis). Numbers of oligodendroglial cells and their molecular markers are reduced. The asymmetry between the hemispheres, which characterises healthy brains, appears reduced in schizophrenia. Dendrites and synaptic markers show alterations. Reduced numbers and reduced functional markers of GABAergic interneurons, particularly in the hippocampus, are a consistent finding in the disorder. (27, pp 286–9, 293)

163. Which of the following statements is most true in family studies of schizophrenia?

    A. Offspring of schizophrenic mothers are at increased risk of schizoid personality disorder.

    B. First-degree relatives of schizophrenic patients are at increased risk of developing bipolar disorder.

    C. First-degree relatives of patients with schizoaffective disorder are at increased risk of schizophrenia but not mood disorder.

    D. There is a clear distinction between genetic factors and the family environment in the aetiology of the disease.

    E. There is unequivocal evidence for a separate genetic transmission of schizophrenia and bipolar disorder.

164. Which of the following statements is most true regarding dementia with Lewy bodies (DLB)?

    A. DLB can be classified as a 'tauopathy'.

    B. DLB has to be considered in patients with REM sleep behaviour disorder.

    C. DLB has neuropathological features that are clearly distinct from Parkinson's disease.

    D. DLB is characterised by deposits of alpha-synuclein, specifically in the basal ganglia.

    E. DLB is characterised by cholinergic hyperactivity in the cerebral cortex.

165. Which of the following statements related to epidemiology is most true?

    A. The term 'inception rate' refers to the number of people who graduate from acutely ill to chronically ill during a defined period.

    B. Cohort studies are carried out in retrospective manner.

    C. Period prevalence describes the number of people who are or have been ill over a defined interval.

    D. The term 'undeclared cases' refers to methodological flaws in the publication of a study.

    E. An odds ratio of 1 generally indicates statistical significance.

166. Which of the following statements is most true related to temporal lobe damage?

    A. Temporal lobe damage results in verbal memory impairment when the right hippocampus is involved.

    B. Temporal lobe damage results in spatial memory impairment when the left hippocampus is involved.

    C. Temporal lobe damage generally does not result in personality changes.

    D. Temporal lobe damage often results in affective symptoms when the right medial temporal lobe is involved.

    E. Temporal lobe damage often results in psychotic symptoms when the right medial temporal lobe is involved.

163. Answer: A. Family studies in schizophrenia clearly indicate a familial aetiology in the disorder. In first-degree relatives of schizophrenic patients, the lifetime risk of developing the disorder is about 5–10%. In addition, the risk for schizotypal, paranoid and schizoid personality disorders is significantly increased. First-degree relatives of patients with schizophrenia have no increased risk of developing bipolar disorder; however, relatives of patients with schizoaffective disorder are at risk of both schizophrenia and bipolar disorder. It is therefore unclear whether there is a separate familial transmission of schizophrenia and mood disorder. Also, family studies do not distinguish between genetic effects and those of the family environment. (27, pp 281–2)

164. Answer: B. Dementia with Lewy bodies (DLB) can be classified as a 'synucleopathy' (as opposed to 'tauopathies' such as Alzheimer's disease) due to the characteristic histopathological feature of aggregated alpha-synuclein in Lewy bodies. Histopathologically, there are no apparent differences between Parkinson's disease and dementia with Lewy bodies. Lewy bodies can be found throughout the cerebral cortex, in the brain stem and in areas of the limbic system. Dementia with Lewy bodies is characterised by widespread loss of choline acetyltransferase (ChAT) in the neocortex and with a resulting cholinergic deficit. Sleep disturbances including REM-sleep behaviour disorder, which is characterised by a loss of the normal inhibition of muscle activity during REM sleep, can be an early clinical characteristic of both DLB and Parkinson's disease. (27, pp 339–40)

165. Answer: C. 'Inception rate' refers to the number of people who are healthy at the beginning of a defined period but became ill during that period. Cohort studies are carried out prospectively on a group of people who are followed for a defined period of time. Period prevalence refers to the number of people who are or have been ill over a defined period of time, as opposed to point prevalence, which describes the number of ill people at a given point in time. The term 'undeclared cases' refers to cases of an illness or condition in the community which are not (yet) known to medical or other agencies. In statistics, an odds ratio of 1 indicates the absence of any differences between two groups. (27, pp 92–3)

166. Answer: D. Widespread temporal lobe damage in the context of dementia, stroke, tumours, epilepsy or trauma can result in a broad-ranging neuropsychiatric clinical pictures, including personality changes. Unilateral temporal lobe lesions produce lateralising deficits. Damage of the left medial temporal lobe is more likely to produce psychotic symptoms, isolated involvement of the left hippocampus results in verbal memory deficits. In contrast, right medial temporal lobe damage is more likely to result in affective changes, and isolated damage of the right hippocampus will produce difficulties with non-verbal (spatial) aspects of memory. (27, p 324)

167. Which of the following statements regarding clomipramine is most true?

   A.   Clomipramine is a selective inhibitor of the re-uptake of 5-HT.
   B.   Clomipramine is less effective than other tricyclic antidepressants in the treatment of obsessive compulsive disorder.
   C.   Clomipramine has been found to have a better antidepressant effect than citalopram and paroxetine in depressed inpatients.
   D.   Clomipramine acts on 5-HT re-uptake via a secondary amine metabolite.
   E.   Clomipramine should reach plasma levels of over 300 ng/mL if the full antidepressant effect is to be achieved.

168. Which of the following statements is most true regarding the brains of severely depressed patients?

   A.   Severely depressed patients brains show increased hippocampal volumes as compared to controls.
   B.   Severely depressed patients brains are characterised by decreased neuronal size and density in the pre-frontal cortex.
   C.   Severely depressed patients brains display regions of diminished white matter intensity on MRI scans.
   D.   Severely depressed patients brains have smaller lateral ventricles than controls.
   E.   Severely depressed patients brains are characterised by up-regulated adult neurogenesis.

169. Which of the following statements about mindfulness-based psychotherapy is most true?

   A.   Mindfulness exploits automatically occurring mental habits.
   B.   Mindfulness actively follows up on and works with internal mental commentary.
   C.   Mindfulness promotes an accepting attitude towards all experience.
   D.   Mindfulness introduces a form of mental conditioning.
   E.   Mindfulness places high importance on the concept of distraction in the therapeutic relationship.

167. Answer: C.

While clomipramine is the most potent tricyclic antidepressant in terms of inhibition of 5-HT re-uptake, it also inhibits noradrenaline re-uptake via its secondary amine metabolite desmethylclomipramine. Studies of depressed inpatients have demonstrated a superior antidepressant effect of clomipramine in comparison with citalopram and paroxetine (Danish University Antidepressant Group, 1990). Clomipramine is also the TCA of choice in the treatment of obsessive compulsive disorder. Similar to other TCAs, total plasma levels should be lower than 300 ng/mL to minimise the risk of toxic side effects such as delirium, seizures and cardiac arrhythmias. (27, p 524)

168. Answer: B.

There are subtle neuropathological changes in patients with severe mood disorders. Lateral ventricles are enlarged (predominantly in elderly subjects with late onset depression), hippocampal volume is decreased (more consistently in unipolar than in bipolar depression). Basal ganglia volume is decreased (in unipolar subjects), volume of the grey matter of subgenual prefrontal cortex is decreased (unipolar and bipolar subjects) and there is increased amygdala volume (bipolar subjects). Cellular pathology includes decreased glial cell numbers (anterior cingulated cortex), decreased neuronal size and density (anterior cingulate and prefrontal cortex) and decreased synaptic markers (pre-frontal cortex). Hyperintense MRI signals of the white matter can be found in subjects with major depression and in normal ageing. The neurotrophic hypothesis of depression is based on the finding that adult neurogenesis, particularly in the hippocampus, is down-regulated in the disorder. (27, pp 242–3)

169. Answer: C.

Mindfulness-based psychotherapy is rooted in Buddhist psychology. Mindfulness is seen as a technique of paying attention in a way that is sensitive, accepting and independent of any thoughts that may be present. In the state of mindfulness, the practitioner may observe automatically occurring mental habits or internal mental commentary, but tries to not actively 'follow up' on these. Instead, an attempt is made to let thoughts pass 'unaltered', and to remain in a state of receptive awareness. In addition, an accepting attitude towards all experience is cultivated. In the therapeutic relationship, mindfulness-based approaches place importance on undistracted attention to the client from the therapist's side. Mindfulness-based therapeutic approaches include mindfulness-based stress reduction (MBSR), mindfulness-based cognitive therapy (MBCT) and dialectical behaviour therapy (DBT), all of which aim in some way to relieve the client from various forms of mental conditioning. (28)

170. Which of the following statements related to disulfiram is most true?

    A.   Disulfiram binds competitively to GABAergic receptors.
    B.   Disulfiram modulates the glutamatergic transmitter system.
    C.   Disulfiram binds to alcohol dehydrogenase.
    D.   Disulfiram leads to increased blood levels of acetaldehyde.
    E.   Disulfiram acts primarily on kidney function.

171. Which of the following statements related to obsessive compulsive disorder (OCD) is most true?

    A.   OCD was first defined by Gilles de la Tourette.
    B.   OCD is associated with childhood infections with *Haemophilus*.
    C.   OCD is characterised by structural abnormalities of the caudate nucleus.
    D.   OCD is evident in as many as 70% of childhood cases with Sydenham's chorea.
    E.   OCD is characterised by 5-HT dysfunction as evidenced by the response to 5-HT re-uptake inhibitors.

172. Which of the following statements related to cognitive analytical therapy (CAT) is most true?

    A.   CAT describes a procedural sequence model that refers to the contents of each therapeutic session.
    B.   CAT holds that faulty procedures are responsible for the low response rate to psychotherapeutic treatments.
    C.   CAT assumes that unrevised maladaptive procedural sequences can help overcome neurotic difficulties.
    D.   CAT postulates that lack of opportunities or neglect in childhood is a main cause for restricted procedural repertoires of the neurotic individual.
    E.   CAT holds that the concept of reciprocal roles unilaterally affects the neurotic individual but not their environment.

170. Answer: E.

Disulfiram inhibits liver aldehyde dehydrogenase, an enzyme critically involved in alcohol metabolism. Any alcohol consumed will lead to increased levels of blood acetaldehyde, exhibiting toxic effects such as facial flushing, nausea, vomiting, gastrointestinal distress, and potentially hazardous hypotension and tachycardia. A different drug used in the treatment of alcohol dependency is acamprosate, which reduces cravings by modulation of the glutamatergic system. Benzodiazepines bind to GABA receptors and are used in alcohol withdrawal. (26, pp 494–5)

171. Answer: D.

Obsessive compulsive disorder has associations with conditions that have known effects on brain function. Up to 70% of childhood cases of Sydenham's chorea have obsessive compulsive symptoms. These symptoms are also associated with Group A streptococcal infections in childhood. While Gilles de la Tourette included obsessional symptoms in his original description of the disorder that now bears his name, he did not define OCD for the first time. Brain imaging studies have revealed no structural abnormalities in OCD, but SPECT and PET studies show increased activity in the orbitofrontal cortex, anterior cingualte, caudate nucleus and parts of the thalamus. 5-HT reuptake inhibitors are an effective treatment of the disorder, but this does not prove that 5-HT function is abnormal. (27, p 198)

172. Answer: D.

Cognitive analytic theory (CAT), developed by Anthony Ryle, is based on the model of procedural sequences. The model supposes that all aim-directed activity is the consequence of an ordered sequence, and unsuccessful adaptation of sequences can lead to 'unrevised maladaptive/faulty procedures', which form the basis for neurotic difficulties. A second cause for difficulties arises from undue restriction in the procedural repertoire, which is caused by impoverished environmental opportunities for learning new procedures. Lack of opportunity can be found in situations of emotional deprivation and neglect, or in childhood abuse of any form. Another important concept in CAT is that of 'reciprocal roles': these internalised role templates are based on early experiences and consist of a role for self, a role for other and a paradigm for their relationship. Examples may include bully/victim, abuser/abused, or caregiver/care receiver. As these role pairs are commonly shared templates, the adoption of one pole by a person will 'pressurise' another interacting person into adopting the congruent pole. The model offers an explanation for the often-difficult patient–therapist dynamics in the context of personality disorders. (29)

173. Which of the following statements about lamotrigine is most true?

    A. Lamotrigine is used as an augmentation agent in patients with refractory depression.

    B. Lamotrigine is started at low doses and increased to the therapeutic dose within two weeks.

    C. Lamotrigine often causes skin rash in patients who have taken it for several months.

    D. Lamotrigine has direct effects on CNS kindling.

    E. Lamotrigine is as effective as lithium in preventing manic episodes in patients with bipolar disorder.

174. In experiments on living patients, which of the following statements about clozapine is most true?

    A. Clozapine has the highest occupancy of striatal D1 receptors of all clinically effective antipsychotics.

    B. Clozapine at higher doses occupies 70–80% of striatal D2 receptors.

    C. Clozapine at low doses only partially occupies cerebral 5-HT2A receptors.

    D. Clozapine dissociates less rapidly from D2 receptors than first-generation antipsychotics.

    E. Clozapine is a potent agonist to 5-HT1A receptors.

175. Which of the following statements regarding anorexia nervosa is most true?

    A. Anorexia nervosa has repeatedly been linked to a polymorphism in the promoter region of the 5HT2A receptor.

    B. Anorexia nervosa affects 5–10% of female siblings of patients with an established anorexic illness.

    C. Anorexia nervosa affects significantly more individuals today than in the 1970s.

    D. Anorexia nervosa affects only 1 male for every 100 females.

    E. Anorexia nervosa has the same concordance rate in monozygotic and dizygotic twin pairs.

173. Answer: A.

The anticonvulsant lamotrigine has been shown to be effective in the prophylactic treatment of mood disorders, particularly rapid cycling bipolar disorder or treatment-resistant depression. In bipolar disorder, lamotrigine is superior to placebo in the prevention of a depressive relapse, but inferior to lithium in the prevention of manic episodes. This has led to its use predominantly in bipolar disorder type II. The most common side effect is skin rash, which is more likely to occur in the initial stages of treatment. A gradual increase of a low starting dose to therapeutic doses (100–200 mg/day) over 1–2 months is recommended to decrease the risk of side effects. Unlike other anticonvulsants, lamotrigine has no direct effect on CNS kindling, a process by which low-level electrical stimulation to certain areas of the brain can lower the seizure threshold. (6, p 197, 26, p 270)

174. Answer: A.

The pharmacological properties of clozapine is complicated, and the exact impacts on the psychopathology of schizophrenic patients have remained unclear. PET and SPECT studies indicate that clozapine has the highest D1 receptor occupancy of all clinically effective antipsychotics. Even at higher doses, clozapine binds only 47–68% of all D2 receptors in the brain. It has been argued that clozapine dissociates more rapidly from D2 receptors than first-generation antipsychotics. Clozapine antagonistically nearly saturates 5-HT2A receptors even at low doses. In contrast, it acts as a partial agonist on 5HT1A receptors. (26, pp 323–4)

175. Answer: B.

Reported incidence rates of anorexia nervosa (AN) in the UK and the U.S. range between 0.37 and 4.06 per 100 000 population per year, and have stayed fairly stable since the 1970s. Of diagnosed patients, 5–10% are males. Family studies suggest a genetic component of the disorder: five to ten per cent of female siblings of patients with established AN will also develop the condition, and monozygotic twins show much higher concordance rates (55%) than dizygotic twins (5%). Association studies have implicated a polymorphism in the promoter region of the 5-HT2A receptor, but this was not replicated in many other investigations. (27, pp 362–3)

176. Which of the following statements about the amnesic syndrome is most true?

    A. The amnesic syndrome is characterised by a circumscribed deficit of speech and reasoning.
    B. The amnesic syndrome is characterised by lack of insight when the medial temporal lobe and the hippocampus are primarily involved.
    C. The amnesic syndrome is characterised by confabulation when the diencephalon is primarily involved.
    D. The amnesic syndrome leads to retrograde amnesia in which more recent events are remembered better than remote events.
    E. The amnesic syndrome leads to abnormal performances on the digit-span test.

177. Which of the following is likely to be least effective in the treatment of antipsychotic-induced akathisia?

    A. Clonazepam
    B. Cyproheptadine
    C. Mirtazapine
    D. Procyclidine
    E. Propranolol

178. Which of the following is thought to best describe the receptor binding of aripiprazole?

    A. Dopamine antagonist
    B. Dopamine partial agonist
    C. Dopamine serotonin antagonist
    D. Glutamate antagonist
    E. Serotonin partial agonist

179. Which of the following is the most suitable treatment for psychosis in a person who has Parkinson's disease?

    A. Aripiprazole
    B. Olanzapine
    C. Quetiapine
    D. Risperidone
    E. Sertindole

180. For which of the following receptors does haloperidol have the greatest affinity?

    A. $Alpha_1$ adrenergic
    B. Dopamine D3
    C. Histamine H_1
    D. Muscarinic cholinergic
    E. Serotonin 5HT3

176. Answer: C.

The amnesic syndrome is characterised by circumscribed and severe deficits in memory function, while global intelligence, speech, reasoning and implicit memory are well preserved. Characteristic features include intact short-term/immediate memory (and intact digit-span test), anterograde amnesia (with severe disturbance of acquisition, retention and recall of verbal and non-verbal material) and retrograde amnesia (with remote events being better remembered than recent events). Based on neuroanatomical distinctions, two subtypes of the syndrome have been described: medial temporal lobe amnesia is characterised by preserved insight, severe anterograde amnesia, limited retrograde amnesia and lack of confabulation. In contrast, diencephalic amnesia (as seen in Korsakoff's syndrome) presents with extensive retrograde amnesia, confabulation and lack of insight. Diencephalic amnesia is attributed to bilateral damage to medial thalamic structures, mammillary bodies and the hypothalamic region. (25, pp 172–3)

177. Answer: D.

Possible measures to treat antipsychotic-induced akathisia are reduction of the antipsychotic dose, change from a first- to a second-generation antipsychotic or treatment with propranolol, low-dose clonazepam, cyproheptadine, mirtazapine, trazodone and mianserin. Diphenhydramine may also help. Anticholinergics are generally ineffective. (6, p 93)

178. Answer: B.

Aripiprazole is thought to differ from most other antipsychotics in that it is a partial agonist at dopamine D2 receptors rather than an antagonist. It is also thought to have 5HT2A antagonist and 5HT1A partial agonist actions (answer E is also true but B best describes the receptor binding). (30, p 422)

179. Answer: C.

Quetiapine has a low propensity to cause extrapyramidal side effects. Other second-generation antipsychotics are more likely to have adverse effects on motor function. First-generation antipsychotics should be avoided in Parkinson's disease. (6, p 426, 30, p 415)

180. Answer: A.

Haloperidol is a dopamine D2 antagonist and also inhibits $alpha_1$ adrenergic receptors. It has little or no affinity for histaminergic or muscarinic cholinergic receptors. (30, p 337)

181. Which of the following is the most common discontinuation symptom on stopping selective serotonin reuptake inhibitor medication?

    A. Concentration and memory difficulties
    B. Hallucinations
    C. Movement disorders
    D. Shock-like sensations
    E. Sweating

182. Which of the following drugs with sedative properties is not a GABA-A-positive allosteric modulator (PAM)?

    A. Flurazepam
    B. Trazodone
    C. Zaleplon
    D. Zolpidem
    E. Zopiclone

183. Which of the following antipsychotic drugs is least likely to cause elevated serum prolactin?

    A. Amisulpride
    B. Clozapine
    C. Olanzapine
    D. Risperidone
    E. Zuclopenthixol

184. Which of the following is least likely to promote wakefulness?

    A. Agomelatine
    B. Caffeine
    C. D-amphetamine
    D. Methylphenidate
    E. Modafinil

185. Which of the following most closely represents the mortality rate of those with neuroleptic malignant syndrome?

    A. 0.5%
    B. 1%
    C. 5%
    D. 10%
    E. 20%

186. Cigarette smoking most likely induces which of the following cytochrome P450 systems?

    A. 1A2
    B. 2D6
    C. 2C9
    D. 2C19
    E. 3A4

181. Answer: D.

Common discontinuation symptoms of SSRIs are influenza like symptoms, shocklike sensations, dizziness, insomnia, irritability and excessive dreaming. Movement disorders can occasionally occur. Sweating and movement disorders can be symptoms of tricyclic antidepressant discontinuation. Occasionally hallucinations occur on discontinuation of monoamine oxidase inhibitors. (6, p 240)

182. Answer: B.

Trazodone is a sedating antidepressant. It is a 5HT2 antagonist, a serotonin reuptake inhibitor, and its sedative actions come from its H1 and $alpha_1$ adrenergic antagonism. The other drugs listed are all GABA-A PAMs. Zaleplon and zolpidem bind selectively to GABA-A receptors that have the α-1 subunit. Benzodiazepines and zopiclone are non-selective and bind to four of the six types of GABA-A α-subunits. (30, pp 839–41, 845)

183. Answer: B.

Clozapine does not exert a significant effect on serum prolactin levels. First-generation antipsychotics, risperidone and amisulpride, have a high propensity to cause elevated serum prolactin. Olanzapine has a minimal effect on serum prolactin. (6, p 10)

184. Answer: A.

Agomelatine may be an effective hypnotic due to its effects as an MT1 and MT2 agonist. (30, p 845)

185. Answer: E.

Neuroleptic malignant syndrome may occur in up to 0.5% of people prescribed antipsychotic medication. It is associated with a mortality rate of approximately 20%. (6, p 11)

186. Answer: A.

Cigarette smoking can induce CYP450 1A2, which metabolises clozapine and olanzapine. Cigarette smokers may require higher doses of these drugs. Conversely, smoking cessation can cause serum levels of drugs to rise. (30, pp 403–4)

187. Which of the following is most likely to have equally prevalent in women and men?

 A. Agoraphobia
 B. Animal phobias
 C. Obsessive compulsive disorder (OCD)
 D. Panic disorder
 E. Social phobia

188. Which of the following best describes the peak incidence of age of onset of OCD?

 A. 14–23 years
 B. 24–34 years
 C. 35–44 years
 D. 45–54 years
 E. 55–64 years

189. Which of the following is most likely a susceptibility gene for ADHD?

 A. ADH2
 B. Apolipoprotein E
 C. BDNF
 D. DRD4
 E. Dysbindin-1

190. Which of the following most closely reflects the risk of bipolar affective disorder in a first degree relative of an affected proband?

 A. 0.5–1%
 B. 5–10%
 C. 15%
 D. 20%
 E. 50%

191. With regard to epilepsy, which of the following is least likely?

 A. A minority of people with epilepsy will develop cognitive impairment.
 B. Higher rates of crime are found in people with epilepsy.
 C. Less than 20% of those with dissociative seizures have a history of epilepsy.
 D. Seventy per cent of people with epilepsy demonstrate epileptiform abnormalities during a first EEG.
 E. Photosensitivity is rare in localisation related epilepsy.

192. Which of the following is most likely to cause teratogenicity?

 A. Carbamazepine
 B. Flurazepam
 C. Lithium
 D. Olanzapine
 E. Sodium valproate

187. Answer: E.

Social phobia is equally prevalent in men and women. All other phobias and anxiety disorders are more common in women. (31, p 195)

188. Answer: B.

The peak incidence for OCD is 24-34 years of age. (31, p 197)

189. Answer: D.

DRD4, DRD5 and DAT1 are thought to be susceptibility genes for the development of ADHD. ADH2 is a susceptibility gene for alcohol dependence, BDNF for bipolar affective disorder, apolipoprotein E for Alzheimer's disease and Dysbindin-1 for schizophrenia. (31, p 46)

190. Answer: B.

Five to ten per cent. This contrasts with 5–10% in population controls. (31, p 47)

191. Answer: D.

Fifty per cent of people with epilepsy demonstrate epileptiform abnormalities on a first routine EEG. Repeated readings will increase the proportion of positive findings. This increases to 80% if a sleep recording is obtained. Approximately a third of those with epilepsy never show an EEG abnormality in an alert state. A generalised spike and wave response to photic stimulation correlates strongly with clinical generalised epilepsy. It is thought that 10–20% of children with epilepsy have impaired intellectual development, with those who have poorly controlled epilepsy being at highest risk. In adults, progressive memory deterioration has been described in up to 50% of those with poorly controlled TLE. There is a higher prevalence of epilepsy among those committed to prison than in the general population. There is no increased prevalence in violent crime, and violence as a consequence of seizures or post-ictal automatisms is rare. (32, p 350)

192. Answer: E.

Valproate is associated with a 7.2% rate of malformations (neural tube defects, facial clefts and cardiac congenital malformations). Carbamazepine has a risk of 2.3% of foetal malformations. Benzodiazepines may carry an increased risk of facial clefts if used in the first trimester. If used in the third trimester they can cause neonatal problems such as floppy baby syndrome. Lithium has a well-documented risk of causing Ebstein's anomaly but the absolute risk is low, 1:1000. Data on the use of olanzapine in pregnancy are limited, but it appears not to be teratogenic. (6, p 370–3)

193. Which of the following models of family therapy focus on hierarchies within families, challenging boundaries and 'unbalancing' family equilibrium?

A. Brief solution-focussed
B. Social constructionist
C. Strategic
D. Structural
E. Systemic

194. A 22-year-old man who has been using cannabis intermittently for five years has been referred by his GP with depressive symptoms. He says that cannabis induces a sense of well-being and sees no point in discontinuing it. Which of the following statements represents the most likely negative outcome of his pattern of drug use?

A. It can produce seizures.
B. It can produce amotivational syndrome.
C. It can cause impairment of short-term memory.
D. Flashbacks of some of the symptoms of intoxication can occur.
E. It can produce visual illusions and hallucinations.

195. Which of the following is most true with regard to the treatment of opiate dependence with methadone?

A. It causes less respiratory depression than buprenorphine.
B. It has milder withdrawal effects than buprenorphine.
C. Untreated withdrawal symptoms reach their peak in 4–6 days.
D. It does not tend to lengthen the QT interval.
E. Opioid withdrawal is a life-threatening condition, which is effectively treated with it.

196. A 25-year-old female asylum seeker who survived stoning for adultery has pushed thoughts of her trauma aside and does not address what happened to her. Which of the following best describes the defence mechanism she is using?

A. Denial
B. Displacement
C. Projection
D. Repression
E. Sublimation

197. Which of the following in relation to subarachnoid haemorrhage (SAH) is least likely?

A. SAH makes up 15% of cerebrovascular incidents.
B. SAH can be precipitated by emotionally stressful events.
C. Two to three per cent of patients will rebleed in the 10 years after surgical clipping.
D. If hydrocephalus occurs, it usually does so in the acute stage after a SAH.
E. Those with autosomal dominant polycystic disease are at high risk.

193. Answer: D.

Salvador Minuchin is associated with the structural school of family therapy. He studied slum families, psychosomatic families and families with a member with an eating disorder. He developed the one-way screen. This is an active approach to family therapy in which dysfunctional alliances are challenged and therapeutic crises are deliberately incited. According to Minuchin, a family is functional or dysfunctional depending on its ability to adapt to different crises. Brief, solution-focused therapy emphasises the competencies of families and individuals. In strategic family therapy the therapist identifies solvable problems, sets goals, designs interventions to achieve these goals and examines the responses. Social constructionist approaches are based on awareness that the observed reality is a creation and the therapists' perceptions are influenced by their own cultures and beliefs. Systemic family therapy was founded in Milan. (31, pp 557–8)

194. Answer: C.

In usual intoxicating doses, cannabis can have both sedative and stimulating effects. It can lead to a sense of well-being, relaxation, a loss of temporal awareness, slowing of cognitive processes and short-term memory impairment. Amotivational syndrome can be a feature of long-term, heavy daily use. Seizures can be a feature of stimulant overdose and benzodiazepine or alcohol withdrawal. Flashbacks, visual illusions and visual hallucinations can occur with hallucinogens such as MDMA and LSD. (30, pp 984–91)

195. Answer: C.

Methadone has a long half-life. Withdrawals reach their peak after 4–6 days, and if untreated, may take 10–12 days to resolve. Untreated heroin withdrawals reach their peak in 32–72 hours after last use and usually subside significantly in 5 days. The opiate partial agonist buprenorphine causes less respiratory depression and milder withdrawal symptoms than methadone. Opioid withdrawal is not an emergency but opioid toxicity is. (6, pp 320–6)

196. Answer: D.

In repression, the person forces a threatening or distressing memory or feeling out of consciousness. Denial involves the failure or refusal to acknowledge some aspect of reality. Displacement involves transferring feelings from their true target onto a harmless substitute. Projection involves displacing one's unacceptable feelings onto someone else. Sublimation involves the diversion of socially unacceptable impulses and drives into socially appropriate, creative ones. (33, p 749)

197. Answer: A.

SAH constitutes approximately 5% of cerebrovascular accidents. (32, pp 491–9)

198. Which of the following noradrenergic receptors is most likely to be pre-synaptic?

A. Alpha 1
B. Alpha 2
C. Alpha 2A
D. Alpha 2B
E. Alpha 2C

199. Regarding cognitive errors in diagnosis, being misled by prototypes is best described by which of the following?

A. Attribution error
B. Availability error
C. Confirmation bias
D. Diagnosis momentum
E. Representative error

200. Which of the following is least true with regard to the epidemiology of Alzheimer's disease?

A. Alzheimer's disease is the most common of the dementias.
B. Rare cases have been reported before the age of 40.
C. People with Asperger's syndrome have a higher risk of developing the disease.
D. The early onset forms occur equally in men and women.
E. Prevalence in the 30–59 age range is 2–3%.

198. Answer: B.

The noradrenaline transporter and alpha 2 autoreceptor are presynaptic. The others listed as well as beta 1, beta 2 and beta 3 are postsynaptic. (30, p 477)

199. Answer: E.

Representative error occurs when a doctor's diagnosis is swayed by prototypes, e.g., misdiagnosing a forty-something farmer's chest pain as a strained muscle because the patient looks too healthy to have heart problems when he actually has unstable angina. The fundamental attribution error is the general tendency to overestimate the importance of personal or dispositional factors relative to situational or environmental factors as causes of behaviour, e.g., if a person does badly in an exam, he or she is more likely to be attributed with having less ability than a student who passed, rather than environmental factors such as illness being taken into account. The availability error determines probability by the ease with which relevant examples come to mind. However, what is available at any given time is often determined by factors that lead to an irrational or erroneous decision, e.g., a doctor who has seen dozens of patients with flulike symptoms during an epidemic may mistakenly misdiagnose another illness as flu. Confirmation bias refers to a type of selective thinking whereby a person tends to notice and to look for what confirms his or her beliefs, and to ignore, not look for or undervalue what contradicts his or her beliefs. For example, if a person believes that during a full moon there is an increase in admissions to hospital, he or she will take notice of admissions during a full moon but be inattentive to the moon when admissions occur during other nights of the month. Diagnosis momentum is the tendency for each doctor brought into a case to accept blindly the initial doctor's diagnosis. (33, p 401, 34)

200. Answer: C.

Alzheimer's disease is the most common of the dementias occurring in 60% of dementia cases. At all ages, women outnumber men by 2 or 3: 1 except in the early onset familial forms of the disease, which have equal prevalence in women and men (autosomal dominant). Prevalence rises exponentially with age and it affects 11% of those aged 80–89 years. People with Down's syndrome have an increased risk of the disease. (32, p 545)

References

1. Puri BK, Tyrer PJ. *Sciences Basic to Psychiatry*. Edinburgh; New York: Churchill Livingstone; 2000.
2. Preskorn SH. Clinically relevant pharmacology of selective serotonin reuptake inhibitors. An overview with emphasis on pharmacokinetics and effects on oxidative drug metabolism. Clin Pharmacokinet. 1997; **32**(Suppl 1):1–21.
3. Goodnick PJ. Pharmacokinetic optimisation of therapy with newer antidepressants. Clin Pharmacokinet. 1994; **27**(4):307–30.
4. Katzung BG. *Basic & Clinical Pharmacology*. 8th ed. New York: Lange Medical Books/McGraw Hill; 2006.
5. Stein G, Wilkinson G. *Seminars in General Adult Psychiatry*. London: Royal College of Psychiatrists; 1998.
6. Taylor D, Paton C, Kerwin R. *Prescribing Guidelines*. 9th ed. London: Informa Healthcare; 2007.
7. Cohen LM, Tessier EG, Germain MJ, Levy NB. Update on psychotropic medication use in renal disease. Psychosomatics. 2004; **45**(1):34–48.
8. Bilia AR, Gallori S, Vincieri FF. St. John's wort and depression: efficacy, safety and tolerability – an update. Life Sci. 2002; **70**(26):3077–96.
9. Liebermann JA, Murray RM. *Comprehensive Care of Schizophrenia: a textbook of clinical management*. London: Martin Dunitz; 2001.
10. Schneider D, Ravin PD. *Tardive Dystonia*, Medscape 2009. Retrieved 30 May 2015.
11. Woolcott JC, Richardson KJ, Wiens MO *et al*. Meta-analysis of the impact of 9 medication classes on falls in elderly persons. Arch Intern Med. 2009; **169**(21):1952–60.
12. Cassano P, Fava M. Tolerability issues during long-term treatment with antidepressants. Ann Clin Psychiatry. 2004; **16**(1):15–25.
13. Lawlor B. *Revision Psychiatry*. Dublin: MedMedia Ltd; 2001.
14. Puri B, Hall A. *Revision Notes in Psychiatry*. London: Arnold; New York: Oxford Unviersity Press; 1998.
15. Merck Research Laboratories. *The Merck Manual of Diagnosis and Therapy*. 18th ed. Beers M, Porter R, editors. Whitehouse Station, NJ: Merck Research Laboratories; 2006.
16. Swartz MS, Stroup TS, McEvoy JP *et al*. What CATIE found: results from the schizophrenia trial. Psychiatr Serv. 2008; **59**(5):500–6.
17. Rupke SJ, Blecke D, Renfrow M. Cognitive therapy for depression. Am Fam Physician. 2006; **73**(1):83–6.
18. Ahuja N, Cole A. Hyperthermia syndromes in psychiatry. Adv Psychiatr Treat. 2009; **15**(3):181–91.
19. American Psychiatric Association. *Diagnostic and Statistical Manual of Mental Disorders: DSM-IV-TR*. Washington, DC: American Psychiatric Association; 2000.
20. Jones I, Smith S. Puerperal psychosis: identifying and caring for women at risk. Adv Psychiatr Treat. 2009; **15**(6):411–8.
21. Stein G, Wilkinson G. *Seminars in General Adult Psychiatry*: London: RCPsych Publications; 2007.
22. Jefferies K, Agrawal N. Early-onset dementia. Adv Psychiatr Treat. 2009; **15**(5):380–8.
23. Morris J. Interpersonal psychotherapy – a trainee's ABC? Psychiatr Bull. 2002; **26**(1):26–8.
24. World Health Organization. *The ICD-10 Classification of Mental and Behavioural Disorders: clinical descriptions and diagnostic guidelines*. Geneva: World Health Organization; 1992.
25. Thambirajah MS. *Psychological Basis of Psychiatry*. Edinburgh; New York: Churchill Livingstone; 2005. pp. 126–7.
26. King D, editor. *Seminars in Clinical Psychopharmacology*. London: Royal College of Psychiatrists, Gaskell; 2004.
27. Gelder M, Cowen P, Harrison P. *Shorter Oxford Textbook of Psychiatry*. Oxford; New York: Oxford University Press; 2006.
28. Mace C. Mindfulness in psychotherapy: an introduction. Adv Psychiatr Treat. 2007; **13**(2):147–54.
29. Denman C. Cognitive–analytic therapy. Adv Psychiatr Treat. 2001;**7**(4):243–52.
30. Stahl S. *Stahl's Essential Psychopharmacology*. 3rd ed. Cambridge; New York: Cambridge University Press; 2008.
31. Wright P, Stern J, Phelan M. *Core psychiatry*. 2nd ed. Philadelphia, PA: Elsevier Press; 2005.
32. David A, Fleminger S, Kopelman M *et al*., editors. *Lishman's Organic Psychiatry*. 4th ed. Chichester, UK: Wiley-Blackwell; 2009.
33. Gross R. *Psychology: the science of mind and behaviour*. London: Hodder Arnold; 2005.
34. *The Skeptic's Dictionary*; 2009. http://www.skepdic.com. Retrieved on the 9th of April 2009.

chapter 03

100 MCQs from Dr. David Browne and Colleagues

Dr Karen Fleming; Dr Michael Kenewali; Dr Manas Sarkar; and Dr Daniel White

201. You are giving a lecture to medical students about genetic factors and their role in influencing susceptibility to various psychiatric disorders. The current evidence most strongly favours dysbindin (DTNBP1) as a susceptibility gene for which one of the following psychiatric disorders?

A. Anorexia nervosa
B. Bulimia nervosa
C. Emotionally unstable (borderline) personality disorder
D. Generalised anxiety disorder
E. Schizophrenia

202. A 79-year-old woman diagnosed with a depressive episode attends your clinic and is receiving antidepressant treatment with citalopram. On review today she complains of muscle cramps, nausea, dizziness and lethargy. She has recently been prescribed ibuprofen by her GP for back pain. Which of the following clinical states most closely fits the symptoms described by this patient?

A. Delirium
B. Hyperkalaemia
C. Hyponatraemia
D. Neuroleptic malignant syndrome
E. Serotonin syndrome

203. Which of the following antidepressants is least likely to cause sedation?

A. Dosulepin
B. Doxepin
C. Mianserin
D. Mirtazapine
E. Reboxetine

204. Which of the following drugs is most likely to induce cytochrome P4502C?

A. Carbamazepine
B. Cimetidine
C. Fluoxetine
D. Fluvoxamine
E. Phenytoin

201. Answer: E.

Much work has been done to identify susceptibility genes in schizophrenia and bipolar disorder. The current evidence implicates specific genes in both disorders. Evidence supports neuregulin 1 (NGR1), dysbindin (DTNBP1), DISC1, D-amino acid oxidase activator (DAOA (G72)), D-amino acid oxidase (DAO) and regulator of G-protein signalling (RGS4) as schizophrenia susceptibility loci. For bipolar disorder the strongest evidence supports DAOA (G72) and brain-derived neurotrophic factor (BDNF). Increasing evidence suggests an overlap in genetic susceptibility across the traditional classification system that dichotomised psychotic disorders into schizophrenia or bipolar disorder, most notably with association findings at DAOA (G72), DISC1, and NGR1. (1, p 572)

202. Answer: C.

This woman presents with symptoms that are associated with hyponatraemia. She has several risk factors for hyponatraemia including being female, elderly and receiving co-therapy with a non-steroidal anti-inflammatory drug (NSAID). While she could have delirium as a consequence of hyponatraemia, this vignette does not describe symptoms associated with delirium such as confusion. Symptoms of serotonin syndrome could include restlessness, diaphoresis, tremor, shivering, myoclonus, confusion or convulsions leading to death. Symptoms of hypokalaemia could include muscle weakness, hypotonia, cardiac arrhythmias, cramps and tetany; they are often due to diuretics. The symptoms of neuroleptic malignant syndrome include fever, diaphoresis, rigidity, confusion, fluctuating consciousness, fluctuating blood pressure, tachycardia, elevated creatinine kinase, leucocytosis and altered liver function tests. (2, pp 210–1, 235, 103–5)

203. Answer: E.

Dosulepin, doxepin and mirtazapine are associated with a high incidence of sedation; mianserin is moderately sedating, and reboxetine is associated with a low incidence of sedation. (2, p 250)

204. Answer: E.

Carbamazepine induces CP4501A2, CP4502D6 and CP4503A. CP4502C is inhibited by cimetidine, fluoxetine and fluvoxamine. Phenytoin induces CP4502C. (2, p 248)

205. Which of the following psychotropic drugs is most extensively metabolised by the liver?

A. Amisulpride
B. Aripiprazole
C. Gabapentin
D. Lithium
E. Sulpiride

206. Which of the following antidepressants is least likely to cause postural hypotension?

A. Fluoxetine
B. Lofepramine
C. Reboxetine
D. Trazodone
E. Venlafaxine

207. You are asked to assess a 63-year-old man by the medical team. He is an inpatient in a medical ward and was diagnosed with an acute myocardial infarction on admission 10 days ago. He is medically stable and ready for discharge from hospital. You find him to be significantly depressed and to require treatment with antidepressant medication. Given the recent myocardial infarction, which of the following antidepressants would you consider most safe in managing this man's depressive illness?

A. Citalopram
B. Duloxetine
C. Fluoxetine
D. Nortriptyline
E. Sertraline

208. Which of the following psychotropic agents are reported to most likely decrease Prothrombin Time/ International Normalised Ratio?

A. Bupropion
B. Carbamazepine
C. Disulfiram
D. Fluoxetine
E. Fluvoxamine

209. A 7-year-old boy diagnosed with attention-deficit hyperactivity disorder (ADHD) is attending your clinic for review. He has been taking methylphenidate for six months with good improvement in his symptoms. His mother reports the emergence of motor tics in the past two weeks and would like a change in her son's medication. Which of the following alternative drug treatments is the most suitable alternative?

A. Atomoxetine
B. Carbamazepine
C. Clonidine
D. Modafinil
E. Risperidone

205. Answer: B.   Aripiprazole is extensively hepatically metabolised. Amisulpride, gabapentin, lithium and sulpiride all undergo no or minimal hepatic metabolism. (2, pp 403–4)

206. Answer: E.   Hypotension is not a problem with venlafaxine, but it can cause increases in blood pressure at higher doses. SSRI antidepressants such as fluoxetine have minimal effect on blood pressure. Reboxetine is associated with marginal increases in both systolic and diastolic blood pressures but may cause a postural decrease in blood pressure at higher doses. Hypotension can be a problem with lofepramine but it is better tolerated than the older tricyclic antidepressants. Trazodone can cause significant decreases in blood pressure. (2, pp 222–4)

207. Answer: E.   Citalopram has been used post–myocardial infarction although license restrictions after myocardial infarction advise caution. Licence restrictions post–myocardial infarction advise caution with duloxetine and although clinical experience with fluoxetine is limited, it is probably safe post–myocardial infarction. Tricyclic antidepressants such as nortriptyline are contraindicated post–myocardial infarction. Sertraline is safe to use post–myocardial infarction and is the drug treatment of choice in this scenario. (2, pp 224–5)

208. Answer: B.   Bupropion, disulfiram, fluoxetine and fluvoxamine have been reported to increase prothrombin time/international normalised ratio. Carbamazepine has been reported to decrease Prothrombin Time/ International Normalised Ratio. (2, p 486)

209. Answer: A.   Atomoxetine is the most suitable alternative. It may be used as a first-line alternative to stimulants such as methylphenidate and dexamphetamine. It may be suitable for children who develop tics while taking stimulants. Third-line drugs include clonidine and tricyclic antidepressants although very few children should be prescribed these drugs for ADHD alone. There is some evidence to support the efficacy of carbamazepine and no evidence to support the use of second-generation antipsychotics; however, risperidone may have a role in those with moderate learning disability. (2, p 281)

210. You are asked to review a 22-year-old woman at your clinic who is undergoing treatment for schizophrenia. She is taking olanzapine and insists she is stopping the medication immediately as she has gained 10 kg in weight since commencement of treatment 18 months ago. You persuade her to consider a trial of another antipsychotic. Which of the following antipsychotic agents might you prescribe as the best possible alternative given this woman's concern regarding weight gain?

A. Aripiprazole
B. Chlorpromazine
C. Quetiapine
D. Risperidone
E. Zotepine

211. Regarding central serotinergic neurotransmission, which of the following serotonin receptors is most likely to operate presynaptically?

A. 5HT1A
B. 5HT2A
C. 5HT2C
D. 5HT1D
E. 5HTY

212. Which of the following is most true of Wernicke's aphasia?

A. Auditory comprehension is impaired.
B. Dysarthria is common.
C. Grammatical structure of speech is severely disrupted.
D. Melody and intonation of speech are disrupted.
E. Patients are usually aware of their communication problem.

213. Which of the following is most likely a feature of pure word-blindness, alexia without agraphia?

A. A right homonymous hemianopia is almost always present.
B. The patient can read what he has written.
C. The patient cannot spell out loud.
D. The patient is unable to copy letters of the alphabet.
E. The patient's writing is grossly disrupted.

214. Which of the following is most likely a feature of pure word-deafness, subcortical auditory dysphasia?

A. The patient can repeat words spoken to him.
B. The patient can write to dictation.
C. The patient hears words as sounds but fails to recognise these sounds as words.
D. The patient's speech is grossly disrupted.
E. The patient's writing is abnormal.

210. Answer: A. Although all antipsychotics may cause weight gain, mean weight gain is highly variable between agents and not all individuals gain weight while taking them. Aripiprazole has a low relative risk of weight gain. Chlorpromazine, quetiapine and risperidone carry a moderate relative risk of weight gain. Zotepine has a moderate or high relative risk of weight gain. (2, p 110)

211. Answer: D. In addition to the serotonin transporter, the 5HT1D receptor is a key presynaptic serotonin receptor and another key presynaptic serotonin receptor is the alpha 2 noradrenergic heteroreceptor. A, B, C and E are all postsynaptic serotonin receptors. (3, p 172)

212. Answer: A. In Wernicke's aphasia auditory comprehension is always impaired. There is no dysarthria; this is in contrast to Broca's aphasia. Speech lacks nouns and verbs, which convey information, although grammatical construction is relatively well preserved. Melody and intonation of speech are preserved. Patients are usually not aware of their problem with communication. (4, p 57)

213. Answer: A. A right homonymous hemianopia is almost invariably present. The patient can write spontaneously and to dictation but subsequently cannot comprehend his or her own written output. The patient can spell out loud and recognises words spelt out loud. The patient, while being unable to recognise letters, can still describe or copy them. The writing is usually entirely normal. (5, p 50)

214. Answer: C. The defect is restricted to the understanding of spoken speech. The patient hears words as sounds but fails to recognise these sounds as words. As a consequence, the patient is unable to repeat words spoken to him/her and cannot write to dictation. The patient can speak fluently and write normally. (5, pp 49–50)

215. Regarding the benzodiazepine drug diazepam, which of the following statements is least likely to be true?

    A. Bioavailability following oral administration is almost complete.
    B. Diazepam is highly lipid soluble.
    C. Elimination is largely via hepatic metabolism.
    D. Following oral administration, peak plasma concentrations are usually reached in 10 minutes.
    E. The elimination half-life is age dependent.

216. Following administration of electroconvulsive therapy (ECT), which of the following acute hormonal changes would most likely be observed?

    A. Adrenocorticotropic hormone (ACTH) falls
    B. Insulin falls
    C. Oxytocin rises
    D. Thyroid-stimulating hormone (TSH) falls
    E. Thyrotropin-releasing hormone (TRH) rises

217. Which of the following statements regarding lithium is most true?

    A. A serum peak level is reached 12 hours after ingestion.
    B. Lithium is absorbed rapidly from the upper gastrointestinal tract.
    C. Lithium is extensively metabolised by the liver.
    D. In terms of pharmacokinetic profile lithium is bound to serum proteins.
    E. There is poor correlation between serum levels and side effects.

218. Which of the following antipsychotic medications is least likely to cause prolactin elevation?

    A. Amisulpride
    B. Chlorpromazine
    C. Clozapine
    D. Risperidone
    E. Sulpiride

219. A 52-year-old woman with a diagnosis of schizophrenia attends your clinic. She is concerned that she has developed abnormal orofacial movements in the preceding month. She is not distressed by them but would like them to stop. She has been prescribed amisulpride 600 mg for many years, and procyclidine 5 mg daily, the indications for which are unclear. You diagnose tardive dyskinesia and find no evidence of other extrapyramidal side effects. Which of the following steps would you be most likely to consider first in an attempt to manage her side effects?

    A. Commence clonazepam 1 mg/day
    B. Commence tetrabenazine 25 mg/day
    C. Commence vitamin E 400–1600 IU/day
    D. Increase procyclidine to 10 mg daily
    E. Reduce the dose of amisulpride

215. Answer: D. Bioavailability following oral dosing of the drug is almost complete and peak plasma levels are usually attained after 30–90 minutes. The rate but not the extent of absorption is reduced by the presence of food. Intramuscular administration is best avoided as absorption is erratic and often slower than following oral administration. (6, p 113)

216. Answer: C. In the acute phase following administration of ECT, adrenocorticotropic hormone, insulin and thyroid-stimulating hormone plasma levels all rise whereas the level of thyrotropin-releasing hormone is not altered by ECT. (6, pp 240–1)

217. Answer: B. A serum peak level is reached 2–3 hours after ingestion. Lithium is not bound to serum proteins, is not metabolised and is excreted unchanged almost entirely by the kidney. There is a good correlation between blood levels and both clinical response and side effects. (6, p 194)

218. Answer: C. In comparison with other antipsychotic medications, clozapine has a very low relative incidence of antipsychotic-induced hyperprolactinaemia. All of the other antipsychotic medications in this question are associated with high relative incidences of antipsychotic-induced hyperprolactinaemia. (2, p 141)

219. Answer: E. Most authorities recommend stopping anticholinergic drugs such as procyclidine as these agents can worsen tardive dyskinesia. You should consider reducing antipsychotic medication, noting that dose reduction may initially worsen tardive dyskinesia. It has now become common practice to withdraw the antipsychotic the individual was taking when tardive dyskinesia was first observed and substitute another drug. Clozapine is best supported in the evidence in this regard; however, there is also support for quetiapine and olanzapine, while there are a few studies supporting risperidone and aripiprazole. Additional drugs are added in if switching antipsychotics is not successful. Tetrabenazine is the only licensed treatment for tardive dyskinesia in the UK. Efficacy for vitamin E is not established. Benzodiazepines may be effective but there are problems with tolerance. (2, pp 92–3, 99)

220. Regarding fragile X syndrome, which of the following statements is most true?

  A. A fragile site on the X chromosome occurs in this syndrome and has been localised to Xq27.
  B. The syndrome affects approximately 0.001% of males.
  C. The syndrome does not occur in females.
  D. The syndrome is a result of an autosomal recessive disorder.
  E. The syndrome is associated with mitral valve prolapse in approximately 20% of cases.

221. Which of the following antidepressant drugs is most likely to prolong the QTc interval on ECG recording at therapeutic doses?

  A. Amitriptyline
  B. Fluoxetine
  C. Mirtazapine
  D. Moclobemide
  E. Venlafaxine

222. Which of the following antipsychotic agents is least likely to prolong the QTc interval on ECG recording at therapeutic doses?

  A. Aripiprazole
  B. Chlorpromazine
  C. Haloperidol
  D. Quetiapine
  E. Sertindole

223. A 35-year-old man with a diagnosis of schizophrenia attends your clinic. He is unable to sit still and constantly crosses and uncrosses his legs. He describes being distressed by subjective restlessness. He is taking quetiapine for treatment of his schizophrenia, which was increased two weeks previously. You diagnose akathisia as a side effect of antipsychotic treatment. Which of the following antipsychotics is an alternative to his current treatment that is least likely to cause akathisia?

  A. Clozapine
  B. Fluphenazine
  C. Haloperidol
  D. Olanzapine
  E. Risperidone

224. You review a 36-year-old married man with a diagnosis of depressive disorder at your clinic. His depressive symptoms have fully resolved following drug treatment with venlafaxine. He now complains of erectile dysfunction. He has read in the patient information leaflet that this may be a side effect of his medication and would like to change to another antidepressant. Which of the following antidepressants is least likely to cause erectile dysfunction?

  A. Citalopram
  B. Fluoxetine
  C. Mirtazapine
  D. Paroxetine
  E. Reboxetine

220. Answer: A. It is the second most common form of intellectual disability after Down's syndrome and affects almost 0.1% of males. Females carrying fragile X sites may demonstrate varying degrees of exophenotypic expression. Mitral valve prolapse occurs in approximately 80% of cases. (7, p 197)

221. Answer: A. Tricyclic antidepressants can prolong the QTc interval at therapeutic doses. When used as single agents, fluoxetine and mirtazapine have no effect on the QTc interval. Moclobemide can prolong the QTc interval following overdose and this is also possible with venlafaxine. (2, p 224)

222. Answer: A. Aripiprazole has no effect on the QTc interval. Chlorpromazine and quetiapine are associated with a moderate effect on QTc. Haloperidol and sertindole are drugs for which extensive QTc prolongation has been noted. (2, pp 117–18)

223. Answer: A. Second-generation atypical antipsychotics have less propensity to induce akathisia compared to older antipsychotics. The following agents are listed in order of decreasing prevalence of akathisia: risperidone, olanzapine, quetiapine and clozapine. (2, pp 92–3)

224. Answer: E. Sexual dysfunction can occur as a side effect of all antidepressants and as part of the clinical picture in depression itself. Individual susceptibility is variable and rates are variable between agents. The approximate prevalence of sexual side effects in treatment with selective serotonin reuptake inhibitors (SSRIs) is 70%. Paroxetine is associated with more erectile dysfunction than other SSRI antidepressants. The approximate prevalence of sexual side effects in treatment with mirtazapine is 25% and is approximately 5–10% with reboxetine. Venlafaxine is estimated to have an approximate prevalence of sexual side effects of 70% with erectile dysfunction being less common. (2, pp 231–2)

225. Which of the following antipsychotics is least likely to cause sedation?

    A. Aripiprazole
    B. Chlorpromazine
    C. Clozapine
    D. Promazine
    E. Zotepine

226. Regarding the pharmacokinetics of psychotropic medication, which of the following is most true?

    A. Drug half-life is inversely proportional to the volume of distribution.
    B. Phase II metabolism is a synthetic reaction.
    C. Steady-state concentration is reached when an equilibrium occurs between absorption and metabolism.
    D. The kidneys preferentially excrete non-ionised compounds.
    E. Water-soluble drugs preferentially cross the blood–brain barrier.

227. In the management of an inpatient presenting with first episode psychosis, which of the following is most correct?

    A. A baseline electrocardiogram (ECG) need only be obtained if the patient has an abnormal physical examination or there is a family history of cardiovascular disease.
    B. Benzodiazepines may be helpful.
    C. Dosages of antipsychotic medication may need to be adjusted according to the patient's weight and gender.
    D. Drug absorption from intramuscular injection is reduced if the patient is agitated.
    E. The addition of a second antipsychotic medication may be helpful if the patient's symptoms persist.

228. Blockade of which of the following receptors is most likely responsible for the reduced sexual dysfunction associated with mirtazapine?

    A. α_1
    B. H_1
    C. $5\text{-}HT_{2c}$
    D. $5\text{-}HT_3$
    E. M_1

225. Answer: A.

In comparison with other antipsychotics, aripiprazole has a very low relative incidence of sedation. All of the other antipsychotics in this question are associated with high relative incidences of sedation. (2, p 141)

226. Answer: B.

Phase II metabolism is a synthetic reaction that converts the active drug to an inactive compound, usually through conjugation with glucuronic acid, rendering it water soluble so that it can be excreted by the kidneys. Drug half-life is directly proportional to volume of distribution. As most psychotropic medications are lipid soluble, their half-lives increase with age as the proportion of adipose tissue increases, leading to an accumulation of the drug in the body. A steady-state concentration is reached when equilibrium occurs between absorption and excretion. The kidneys preferentially excrete ionised and water-soluble compounds. Lipid soluble drugs preferentially cross the blood–brain barrier. (8, pp 32–5)

227. Answer: B.

Alongside antipsychotic medication, benzodiazepines play an important role in the management of aggression when non-pharmacological methods have been unsuccessful. A baseline ECG should be performed on all inpatients presenting with first-episode psychosis, preferably before the commencement of medication. Antipsychotic medication should be commenced at the lowest dose and slowly titrated upwards; larger patients or male patients should not be given higher doses of medication. Drug rate of absorption from intramuscular injection may be significantly increased in patients who are acutely agitated. Polypharmacy should be avoided in patients when possible because of the risks of reduced adherence and increased side effects. If a patient with first-episode psychosis has not adequately responded to an initial trial with an antipsychotic, it should be cross-titrated with a second antipsychotic and stopped. (9, 10)

228. Answer: C.

Blockade of the 5-HT_{2c} receptor is the mechanism through which mirtazapine is associated with a reduction in sexual dysfunction. Blockade of the 5-HT_3 receptor has an anti-nausea effect. Blockade of adrenergic and muscarinic receptors is generally associated with increased sexual dysfunction. The anti-histaminergic effects of mirtazapine are responsible for its sedative properties. (8, p 71)

229. With respect to electro-convulsive therapy (ECT), which of the following is most true?

    A. Bifrontal electrode placement increases the likelihood of cognitive side effects.
    B. Cognitive side effects reduce as ECT treatment progresses.
    C. Low-dose unilateral ECT may be as effective as bilateral ECT.
    D. ECT is moderately effective in the treatment of refractory schizophrenia.
    E. Thirty per cent of patients receiving ECT will relapse within the following year.

230. In a patient who fulfils the diagnostic criteria for treatment-resistant depression and is currently receiving a single antidepressant, which of the following augmentation strategies is most likely to be efficacious?

    A. Adding a second antidepressant
    B. Adding lamotrigine
    C. Adding lithium carbonate
    D. Adding low-dose olanzapine
    E. Adding sodium valproate

231. Regarding psychotherapy, which of the following is most true?

    A. High levels of transference interpretation in sessions may be associated with higher levels of therapeutic alliance.
    B. Drawing the patient's attention to dysfunctional thinking patterns may be helpful if there is a poor therapeutic alliance.
    C. Therapist experience has little effect in the treatment of complicated cases.
    D. The therapeutic alliance makes a modest contribution to outcome.
    E. The therapist's evaluation of the therapeutic alliance in sessions is the best predictor of outcome.

232. Which of the following is least likely a function of the limbic system?

    A. Arousal
    B. Declarative memory
    C. Food intake
    D. Procedural memory
    E. Sexual behaviour

233. Regarding the embryonic development of the central nervous system, which of the following is most true?

    A. Three distinct germ cell layers become apparent during the third week of embryonic development.
    B. The neural tube is completely formed by the end of the second week of embryonic development.
    C. The prosencephalon, mesencephalon and rhombencephalon are identifiable by the fifth week of embryonic development.
    D. The midbrain is derived from the metencephalon.
    E. The cerebral hemispheres develop from the diencephalon.

229. Answer: D.

ECT is usually reserved as a last-line option in the treatment of schizophrenia. It has been found to have a moderate effect in open studies. Its use in schizophrenia is not however recommended in the NICE guidelines. Bifrontal electrode placement has been shown to reduce the likelihood of cognitive side effects when compared with bitemporal electrode placement. Cognitive side effects increase during the course of ECT. High-dose unilateral ECT may be as effective as bilateral ECT. Approximately 50% of patients receiving ECT will relapse within the following 12 months. (2, p 66, 8, pp 74–7)

230. Answer: C.

Although all of the medications listed are useful augmentation strategies for treatment-resistant depression, the evidence for lithium is strongest, with response rates of 50–60%. (11, p 2843)

231. Answer: D.

The therapeutic alliance has been demonstrated in studies to have a small but statistically significant effect on outcome from psychotherapy. The patient's evaluation of the therapeutic alliance is a better predictor of outcome than the therapist's. Attempts to heal rifts in the therapeutic alliance by attributing the patient's feelings to 'dysfunctional thinking patterns' may cause further damage to the therapeutic alliance. Over-reliance on the interpretation of transference, inappropriate self-disclosure and over-structuring sessions are associated with lower levels of therapeutic alliance. Studies suggest that the level of therapist experience and training do not make a significant contribution to outcome except in patients with more complex problems. (12, pp 461–78)

232. Answer: D.

Procedural memory, the ability to perform a previously learned skill (e.g., driving), is a function of the basal ganglia and cerebellum. Declarative memory, the ability to recall facts, is a function of the hippocampus (which is part of the limbic system). The limbic system is also involved in homeostatic behaviour such as arousal in the fight-or-flight reaction, sexual behaviour and food intake. (13, pp 280–95)

233. Answer: C.

The prosencephalon, mesencephalon and rhombencephalon are identifiable by the fifth week of embryonic development. The three germ cell layers of the embryo become apparent at the beginning of the second week of development. The neural tube is fully developed by the end of the fourth week. The midbrain is derived from the mesencephalon. The cerebral hemispheres develop from the telencephalon (the diencephalon gives rise to the thalamus). (14, pp 172–3, 15, pp 4–7)

234. Which of the following diseases is most correctly paired with its macroscopic neuropathology?

A. Creutzfeldt–Jakob disease (CJD): 'knife-blade' atrophy.
B. Huntington's disease: atrophy of the basal ganglia.
C. Parkinson's disease: perforated septum pellucidum.
D. Pick's disease: depigmentation of the substantia nigra.
E. Punch-drunk syndrome: selective cerebellar atrophy.

235. A 55-year-old married woman is referred to your clinic by her general practitioner. Her husband tells you that over the past year she has progressively become less active about the house. Last week she arrived home without the shopping and told her husband that she argued with the checkout operator after she had jumped the queue. She has become verbally aggressive and inappropriate at social events. She scores 28/30 on the Folstein Mini-Mental State Examination, performing poorly on testing of verbal fluency and abstraction. Which of the following diagnoses best fits this clinical picture?

A. Alzheimer's disease
B. Creutzfeldt-Jakob disease (CJD)
C. Huntington's disease
D. Lewy-body dementia
E. Pick's disease

236. Regarding the sequelae of head injury, which of the following is most correct?

A. Twenty per cent of patients will develop cognitive impairment following severe head injury.
B. Thirty per cent of patients will suffer personality change following severe head injury.
C. Ten per cent of patients with penetrating injuries will develop epilepsy.
D. Duration of anterograde amnesia is a poor prognostic indicator.
E. Twenty per cent of patients with impaired consciousness lasting one month will return to work.

237. Which one of the following antipsychotic medications is least likely to prolong the cardiac QT interval?

A. Amisulpride
B. Aripiprazole
C. Olanzapine
D. Quetiapine
E. Risperidone

238. With regard to the epidemiology of suicide, which of the following is most correct?

A. Seventy per cent of people who commit suicide have made previous attempts.
B. Alcohol has been detected in one in six suicides.
C. Suicide rates for people aged 65 years and older have been increasing over previous decades.
D. Suicide risk in depression increases with increasing levels of treatment.
E. The male suicide rate is 50% higher than female suicide rate.

234. Answer: B.

On neuroimaging, atrophy of the basal ganglia, especially in the caudate nucleus, is observed in Huntington's disease. Selective cerebellar atrophy is observed in CJD. Depigmentation of the substantia nigra occurs in Parkinson's disease. A perforated septum pellucidum is a characteristic finding in punch-drunk syndrome and 'knife-blade' atrophy is observed in Pick's disease. (14, pp 193–203)

235. Answer: E.

The presentation is one of personality change, characterised by disinhibition, loss of motivation and irritability suggesting a frontal lobe dementia, consistent with Pick's disease. The absence of an episodic memory deficit makes Alzheimer's disease less likely. (16, pp 162–4)

236. Answer: E.

Only 20% of people who suffer a serious head injury with impaired consciousness lasting one month will be able to re-enter employment. Forty per cent of patients with impaired consciousness lasting one month will die. Three per cent of patients who suffer severe head injuries will experience cognitive impairment, especially if there is a long period of post-traumatic amnesia (greater than 48 hours), there is damage to the left fronto-parietal areas of the brain, and there is a penetrating injury or complications such as haemorrhage or infection occur. Up to 18% of patients will develop personality change, which may occur directly as a result of brain damage or may be an exaggeration of premorbid personality traits. Thirty per cent of patients with penetrating head injuries will develop epilepsy. (17, pp 192–5)

237. Answer: B.

Aripiprazole has been shown to have no effect on QTc interval. Amisulpride, olanzapine and risperidone have all been shown to have a low effect on QTc interval. Quetiapine has a moderate effect on QTc interval. (2, p 117)

238. Answer: D.

The risk of suicide increases with intensity of treatment and a history of inpatient admission, reflecting the fact that patients with severe illness receive higher levels of treatment. Alcohol has been detected in one in three suicides. The suicide rate for the over 65 years of age has progressively fallen over the past two decades. The male suicide rate is 2–4 times the female suicide rate. Up to 40% of suicides have made a previous attempt(s). (18, pp 1033–44)

239. Regarding the genetics of schizophrenia, which of the following statements is most true?

A. Anticipation is frequently reported.
B. Candidate genes such as the D3 gene and the HLA locus on chromosome 6 have been identified as having a weak effect in linkage studies.
C. Cerebral ventricle volume is normal in obligate carriers.
D. Paranoid schizophrenia has a lower monozygotic concordance rate than other types of schizophrenia.
E. There is a higher concordance rate in monozygotic twins with late onset psychosis.

240. Regarding the agnosias, which of the following is most true?

A. Agraphia is a type of agnosia.
B. In the doppelgänger phenomenon, the patient believes the hallucination to be real.
C. Lesions involving the frontal cortex of the brain may be responsible for visual object agnosia.
D. Recognition is composed of perception and identification.
E. The term was first introduced by Freud.

241. An overweight 21-year-old male arts student with a family history of diabetes mellitus has been admitted as a voluntary patient under your care with a two-month history of hearing voices commenting on his actions. He tells you that he believes the children on his street are breaking into his house and rearranging his possessions. He is not aggressive and states that he is happy to remain on the ward. Which of the following statements is most true?

A. Cognitive behavioural therapy is likely to confer significant improvements to his mental state.
B. Cognitive behavioural therapy reduces the likelihood of relapse.
C. If he refuses to take oral medication, he should be detained under the Mental Health Act and given medication intramuscularly.
D. He is likely to become physically aggressive at some point during his admission.
E. Olanzapine would be the antipsychotic medication of choice.

239. Answer: D.

Paranoid schizophrenia has a lower monozygotic concordance rate than other types of schizophrenia. Anticipation is the development of symptoms at younger ages in successive generations. It has been reported in some studies; however most studies have not shown this effect. Candidate genes are used in association studies, where the frequencies of different alleles for a suspect gene (e.g., a dopamine receptor gene) are compared between subjects and controls. Linkage studies look for genetic markers that co-segregate with the disease in high-risk families (those with numerous affected family members). Cerebral ventricular volume is increased in obligate carriers (those without the illness who appear to transmit the liability to the disorder). There is a higher concordance in rate in monozygotic twins with early onset psychosis. (18, pp 599–601)

240. Answer: E.

While the term 'agnosia' was first introduced by Freud, the condition had been described much earlier. The agnosias are a group of disorders characterised by impairments in the recognition of objects. Agraphia is a type of apraxia rather than an agnosia. The doppelgänger phenomenon describes an autoscopic hallucination of the body being projected into external space. It is usually experienced by the patient as being pathological. Recognition is composed of a two-step process – the perception of an object, followed by the association of the object with meaning. While many agnosic patients experience a combination of deficits in the areas of apperception and association, some have agnosias that are either apperceptive or associative, e.g., the apperceptive agnosic cannot copy a drawing whereas the associative agnosic can copy the drawing but cannot identify it. Lesions of the occipital, parietal and temporal regions of the brain are responsible for visual object agnosia. (5, pp 58–60)

241. Answer: A.

Cognitive behavioural therapy (CBT) has been shown to significantly reduce psychopathology compared with standard treatment in the early stages of psychosis and leads to significantly shorter inpatient admissions. While CBT in this group of patients does not reduce relapse rates, patients exhibit fewer positive symptoms in subsequent presentations. Verbal aggression is common in patients admitted with a first episode of psychosis, physical violence is not. The association between olanzapine and glycaemic dysregulation would suggest that an alternative antipsychotic medication should be used in this man who is at an increased risk of diabetes mellitus. (12, p 286, 19)

242. Regarding memory, which of the following is most correct?

 A. Amnesic patients perform poorly in tests of priming compared to normal controls.
 B. Implicit memory is preserved in amnesic patients.
 C. In the early stages of illness, memory is more impaired in Pick's disease compared with vascular dementia.
 D. Recall of day-to-day events is impaired in patients with semantic dementia.
 E. The question 'what colour is a fire engine?' is a test of declarative memory.

243. Regarding the epidemiology of affective disorders, which of the following is most correct?

 A. Dysthymia typically starts in middle age.
 B. Individuals with more than one medical condition are twice as likely to suffer a severe depressive episode.
 C. Mania presents with psychotic symptoms in approximately 10% of cases.
 D. Unipolar mania is equally common among males and females.
 E. Women with bipolar affective disorder are more likely to suffer a depressive episode than men.

244. Regarding the treatment of substance use disorders, which of the following is most correct?

 A. A short course of benzodiazepines may assist the symptomatic treatment of opiate withdrawal.
 B. Disulfiram inhibits the alcohol dehydrogenase enzyme.
 C. Methadone in tablet and sugar-free preparations is less likely to be injected.
 D. Evidence for the efficacy of naltrexone in the treatment of alcohol dependence is limited.
 E. Pregnant women should be withdrawn from opiates immediately.

245. Regarding the treatment of catatonia, which of the following is most true?

 A. Antipsychotic medications may be helpful in the acute stages of treatment.
 B. Approximately 50% of patients may require electroconvulsive therapy.
 C. Lethal catatonia may be distinguished from neuroleptic malignant syndrome upon clinical examination and laboratory investigation.
 D. Lorazepam doses of up to 24 mg should be used before electroconvulsive therapy is considered.
 E. Patients with comorbid schizophrenia or mood disorders have similar response rates to treatment.

242. Answer: B.

Implicit memory, a function of the basal ganglia, is preserved in amnesic patients. Priming, the 'subconscious' influence of previous learning on a task, is a feature of implicit memory. Memory is relatively preserved in the early stages of Pick's disease compared with vascular dementia and Alzheimer's disease. Semantic memory is the ability to recall factual information. In semantic dementia, also known as Pick's disease in which there is focal temporal lobe involvement, there is a selective loss of factual knowledge, e.g., what is the colour of a fire engine? Orientation and episodic memory, and memory of day-to-day events are substantially preserved in semantic dementia. (16, pp 16–19)

243. Answer: E.

Women are over-represented in all groups of affective disorders where depression is a major component, including bipolar affective disorder subgroups such as rapid cycling and bipolar type II disorder. Dysthymia typically begins in late adolescence or early adulthood. Mania presents with psychotic symptoms in approximately 20% of cases. Males are significantly over-represented in unipolar mania. (11, pp 1575–81)

244. Answer: A.

A short course of benzodiazepines may assist the symptomatic treatment of opiate withdrawal. Disulfiram acts by inhibiting the aldehyde dehydrogenase enzyme, resulting in an accumulation of acetaldehyde in the blood and the experience of unpleasant symptoms such as headaches, nausea and palpitations. Alcohol dehydrogenase is the enzyme that converts ethanol to acetaldehyde. Methadone is more likely to be injected in tablet or sugar-free preparations. Naltrexone has been shown to reduce cravings and relapse rates in alcohol-dependent subjects. It is a safe and moderately effective treatment according to results in a Cochrane meta-analysis. Sudden withdrawal from opiates may result in spontaneous abortion. (14, pp 348–56, 20)

245. Answer: D.

Approximately 80% of patients with catatonia will respond to standard doses of lorazepam; however, doses of up to 24 mg may be required before ECT is considered. Malignant catatonia and NMS are indistinguishable from each other and NMS is thought to be a variant of malignant catatonia. Antipsychotic medications are therefore best avoided in the acute phases of catatonia, particularly malignant catatonia. Patients with comorbid schizophrenia have a poorer response to treatment of catatonia compared with those with bipolar disorder. (2, pp 106–7)

246. A 29-year-old married woman with bipolar affective disorder attends her routine psychiatric outpatient appointment with her husband. She is in her fourth week of pregnancy according to her general practitioner. She asks your advice about the safety of continuing lithium. Her last episode of mania was nine months ago. Which of the following is most correct?

A. Lithium should be discontinued immediately.
B. If the withdrawal of lithium results in relapse, sodium valproate, carbamazepine or lamotrigine may be helpful as alternative mood stabilisers.
C. She should have an urgent ultrasound to screen for Ebstein's anomaly.
D. Lithium should be continued throughout the pregnancy.
E. Breastfeeding is contraindicated if she remains on lithium during the post-natal period.

247. Regarding the treatment of obsessive compulsive disorder, which of the following is most correct?

A. Cognitive and behavioural strategies are more effective than serotonergic antidepressants.
B. Group therapy is less effective than individual therapy.
C. Ten to fifteen per cent of patients believe their obsessional thoughts are rational.
D. More frequent therapy sessions are associated with improved outcomes.
E. Treatment of any kind is more successful if compulsions are present.

248. Regarding caregiver burden in dementia, which of the following is most correct?

A. Depressive symptoms are reported less frequently among female caregivers.
B. Mortality rates of people experiencing caregiver strain are 60% higher than non-caregivers.
C. White caregivers report fewer symptoms of psychological distress than caregivers of other races.
D. Psychological distress in the caregiver is reduced when a patient with dementia is admitted to long-term care.
E. Approximately 20% of caregivers suffer with depression.

249. With respect to the electroencephalogram (EEG), triphasic waves are least likely to be present in which of the following?

A. Alzheimer's disease
B. Anoxic brain damage
C. Creutzfeldt–Jakob disease
D. Hepatic encephalopathy
E. Huntington's disease

246. Answer: E.

Breastfeeding is a relative contraindication due to reports of neonatal toxicity and is generally advised against if the mother is receiving lithium. The recommendations in pregnancy are that lithium be withdrawn slowly prior to conception, to reduce the risk of relapse. If the withdrawal of lithium is unsuccessful, it should be recommenced and the risks to the foetus should be discussed with the patient. Other mood stabilisers such as sodium valproate, carbamazepine and lamotrigine are associated with higher risks of congenital malformation and should be avoided if possible. High-resolution (level 2) ultrasound and echocardiography are recommended at weeks 6 and 18 of gestation if the patient remains on lithium. The risk of Ebstein's anomaly is around 1:1000 and is greatest in the first trimester. (2, pp 383–4)

247. Answer: E.

Treatment is more effective if compulsions are present. Cognitive and behavioural therapies have similar effectiveness to SSRIs. Likewise, group and individual therapies have similar success rates. Up to a third of patients in one study believed that their obsessional thoughts were rational. Patients with more bizarre obsessional thoughts are less likely to resist carrying out compulsive acts. The frequency of psychotherapy sessions has not been shown to influence outcome although duration of each session and the therapy overall is associated with better outcomes. (12, pp 198–215)

248. Answer: B.

Compared with non-caregivers and caregivers who do not report strain associated with caregiving, caregivers reporting strain have an increased mortality rate of approximately 60% higher. This may be due to the physical effects of chronic stress and self-neglect associated with caring for a patient with dementia. Females are more likely to report depressive symptoms. Non-white caregivers use a variety of coping mechanisms such as religion and have strong beliefs of family responsibility, hence the reduced level of distress experienced in the care of these patients. Levels of psychological distress among caregivers as a group have been shown to be relatively stable over time. While admitting a relative with dementia to a care facility may reduce distress in some cases; feelings of guilt and sadness have been reported in those who had relatives placed in nursing homes. At least 30% of caregivers report symptoms of depression while caring for a family member with dementia. (11, p 3841)

249. Answer: E.

Huntington's disease is associated with pronounced flattening of the EEG record with a virtual absence of rhythmic activity. (5, p 131, 14, p 541)

250. A 3-year-old boy is referred to a child psychiatrist with deficits in attention, motor control and perception. The psychiatrist suspects the presence of DAMP (deficits in attention, motor control and perception). Which of the following is the most relevant in developmental history-taking?

A. Excess maternal iron intake
B. Excess maternal alcohol intake
C. Hormonal treatment
D. Maternal heroin intake
E. Rubella vaccination

251. A patient with schizophrenia presents to his GP with frequent urination, excessive thirst, hunger and weight loss. He has been taking olanzapine 20 mg for the last year. His GP suspects that he might have developed diabetes. What is the most likely odds ratio for developing diabetes on olanzapine compared to controls not taking antipsychotic medications?

A. 1–2
B. 2–3
C. 4–6
D. 10
E. None of the above

252. A 24-year-old Caucasian man with a history of paranoid schizophrenia was found by his parents in a lethargic state. He has a history of suicide attempts and admitted to ingesting 2000 mg quetiapine. Which of the following is the least likely to be observed in quetiapine overdose?

A. Heart block
B. Chest pain
C. Hypocalcaemia
D. Myocarditis
E. QT prolongation

253. A 19-year-old girl with bulimia nervosa on fluoxetine medication asks her psychiatrist for psychotherapy. Of the following psychological therapies available for a person with an eating disorder, which would be the most likely to be applicable?

A. Art therapy
B. Cognitive behavioural therapy
C. Family dialectical behavioural therapy
D. Music therapy
E. Nidotherapy

254. A 44-year-old man recovering from a road traffic accident complained he found it difficult to find his way around both familiar and new places. Injury to which part of the brain is most likely to cause this sort of a symptom?

A. Cerebellar injury
B. Frontal lobe injury
C. Optic chiasm injury
D. Right parietal lobe injury
E. Temporal lobe injury

250. Answer: B. The concept of DAMP (deficits in attention, motor control and perception) has been in clinical use in Scandinavia for about 20 years. DAMP is diagnosed on the basis of concomitant attention deficit/hyperactivity disorder and developmental coordination disorder in children who do not have severe learning disability or cerebral palsy. In clinically severe forms, it affects about 1.5% of the general population of school-age children. Boys are overrepresented; however this may be because girls are underdiagnosed. Maternal alcohol abuse in pregnancy appears to be associated with a much increased risk of DAMP in the offspring. Equally, smoking in pregnancy probably has a separate effect on the odds for developing DAMP or ADHD in the child. (21)

251. Answer: D. The UK General Practice Research Database compared 451 new incident cases of diabetes with 2696 controls not on antipsychotic medication. The odds ratio was 5.8 for the risk of developing diabetes for patients taking olanzapine compared with controls. (22)

252. Answer: B. Haloperidol and other typical antipsychotics are known to cause cardiac conduction abnormalities, including QTc interval prolongation on electrocardiogram (ECG). Atypical antipsychotics such as olanzapine, risperidone and quetiapine have a reputation for cardiovascular safety. Quetiapine overdose can cause cardiac anomalies and there are several case reports of this finding in the Academy of Psychosomatic Medicine. (23)

253. Answer: B. Quite a few forms of psychological treatment are available for bulimia. The most commonly used is cognitive behavioural therapy. Dialectical behavioural therapy and family therapy have also been widely used. For anorexia nervosa, apart from psychodynamic therapy and family therapy, the Maudsley Clinic have their own Maudsley approach. (24)

254. Answer: D. The parietal lobe is located just behind the frontal lobe. Damage to the right parietal lobe can cause visuospatial deficits, e.g., the patient may have difficulty finding his or her way around both familiar and new places. Damage to the left parietal lobe area can result in disruption in the patient's ability to understand written or spoken language. (25)

255. The Rancho Los Amigos Scale (RLAS) is useful in assessing the patient in the first weeks or months following a brain injury as it does not require cooperation from the patient. Which of the following measures are RLAS levels based on?

   A. Blood pressure
   B. Electrocardiogram findings
   C. Pupillary response
   D. Response to external stimulus
   E. Skin sensitivity

256. Which of the following statements is most true?

   A. Acetylcholine is an inhibitory transmitter and is implicated in Alzheimer's disease.
   B. Dopamine is a inhibitory neurotransmitter involved in bipolar affective disorder.
   C. Gamma-amino butyric acid is an excitatory neurotransmitter that is implicated in schizophrenia.
   D. Only axons that have myelin sheaths can carry signals.
   E. Serotonin is an inhibitory transmitter that constricts blood vessels and brings on sleep.

257. Which of the following is least likely to be a side effect of treatment with methylphenidate medication?

   A. Exacerbation of tics
   B. Erythema multiforme
   C. Insomnia
   D. Palpitations
   E. Weight gain

258. Which one of the following genes is most likely to be implicated in attention-deficit hyperactivity disorder (ADHD)?

   A. Dopamine active transporter gene (DAT-1)
   B. RNA gene
   C. *E. coli* gene
   D. Transposon
   E. HCV gene

255. Answer: D.

The Rancho Los Amigos Scale (RLAS) is most helpful in assessing the patient in the first weeks or months following a brain injury because it does not require cooperation from the patient. The RLAS is based on observation of the patient's response to external stimuli. The RLAS provides a descriptive guideline of the various stages a brain injury patient will experience as they progress to recovery. (26, pp 511–12)

256. Answer: E.

Serotonin is an inhibitory neurotransmitter that constricts blood vessels and brings on sleep and is involved in temperature regulation. Dopamine is an inhibitory neurotransmitter involved in mood and the control of complex movements. The loss of dopamine activity in some portions of the brain leads to the muscular rigidity of Parkinson's disease. Many medications used to treat behavioural disorders work by modifying the action of dopamine in the brain. (27)

257. Answer: E.

Decreased appetite is common but usually transient. Nervousness and insomnia are the most common adverse reactions reported with methylphenidate. They are usually controlled by reducing dosage and omitting the drug in the afternoon or evening. Central nervous system adverse effects are dizziness, drowsiness, headache and dyskinesia. Other side effects include hyperactivity, convulsions, muscle cramps, choreo-athetoid movements, tics (exacerbation of pre-existing tics) and Tourette's syndrome. Psychotic episodes, including hallucinations, which subsided when methylphenidate was discontinued, have been reported. Although a definite causal relationship has not been established, isolated cases of transient depressed mood as well as symptoms of visual disturbances on rare occasions have been described. Difficulties with accommodation and blurring of vision have also been noted. (28, pp 1002–3)

258. Answer: A.

Meta-analysis of genetic data in IMpACT has so far focused mainly on established ADHD genes from studies in children. The gene encoding the dopamine transporter DAT1, a regulator of signalling through the neurotransmitter dopamine in the brain, has been studied multiple times. Though results have been inconsistent for single genetic variants, a combination of genetic variations at two positions of the gene seems to increase ADHD risk in children. However, in a recent study of 1440 patients and 1769 controls in IMpACT, a different combination of variants at the same two positions was found to increase the risk for the persistent adult form of ADHD. This shows that age is an important factor to be taken into account in genetic association studies in ADHD and might explain some of the discrepancies in earlier studies. Transposons are sequences of DNA that can transpose into new positions in the genome of a single cell. (29)

259. Which of the following would be the most effective measure to check out the prevalence of schizophrenia in a given population?

    A. Audit
    B. Cross-sectional survey
    C. Cohort study
    D. Case–control study
    E. Randomised control study

260. With regard to statistical measures, which of the following best describes 'number of children'?

    A. Binary measure
    B. Continuous measure
    C. Ratio measure
    D. Dichotomous variable
    E. Quantitative variable

261. Which of the following is most likely to be a neuronal secretory product of specialised hypothalamic neuroendocrine transducer cells that convert a neural impulse into a hormone?

    A. Fatty acid
    B. Neurohormone
    C. Peptide
    D. Steroid
    E. Thyroid hormone

262. There are mainly three levels of epidemiological investigations, namely analytical, descriptive and experimental. Which one of the following best describes an analytical study?

    A. Assessing individual risks
    B. Completing the clinical picture
    C. Community diagnosis
    D. Identifying causes
    E. Identification of syndromes

263. With regards to epidemiology, which of the following statements is most true?

    A. Lifetime prevalence is almost always based on subject recall, which can be inaccurate.
    B. Lifetime prevalence rate does allow for the fact that incidence rates might have changed.
    C. Lifetime prevalence is a standard and not a measure.
    D. Lifetime prevalence includes those over the represented full age range.
    E. Lifetime prevalence is used to summarise the number of cases of a disorder that exist at any time during a specified time period.

259. Answer: B.   A cross-sectional study is generally used to look at the prevalence of an illness in a given population. All the members of the population are surveyed for a particular illness. They are generally useful for planning services, drawing public attention to a particular problem, making comparisons with other populations and charting trends over time. (30, p 121)

260. Answer: E.   'Number of children' should be considered as a discrete quantitative variable. Continuous variables are measures of attributes that can be indexed at any point along a scale. Quantitative variables are sometimes referred to as ordinal scales. (30, p 116)

261. Answer: B.   Neurohormones are neuronal secretory products of specialised hypothalamic cells. They are released from the median eminence into the portal hypophyseal bloodstream and carried to the pituitary to regulate the release of anterior pituitary hormones. They are in essence any hormones released by a neuron. (31, pp 104–5)

262. Answer: A.   Analytical studies are those that explore the basis of variations in illness rates among different groups in order to identify risk factors that may contribute to the development of the disorder. Once the basic rates of illness are established, it is possible to identify groups in the population with high rates of illness. (31, pp 378–9)

263. Answer: A.   Lifetime prevalence is a measure of the number of individuals who at some point in their life had the illness under study. It may be used to describe the overall occurrence of a remittent disease (arthritis) in a population. (31, pp 384–5)

264. A polymorphism can be detected using polymerase chain reaction (PCR). Which of the following is least true about PCR markers?

    A. They are abundant.
    B. They spread evenly throughout the genome.
    C. They have heterozygosity values that average from 60% to 90%.
    D. They selectively amplify small regions of the genome.
    E. They rely on Southern blot analysis.

265. Which one of the following is least likely to be included in the 'metapsychological concepts' that form the foundation of the psychoanalytical theory of mental phenomenon?

    A. Dynamic
    B. Economic
    C. Equilibrium
    D. Genetic
    E. Topographical

266. Which one of the following is least likely to be a side effect of paroxetine treatment?

    A. Agitation
    B. Constipation
    C. Chronic pain
    D. Shortening of left ventricular ejection time
    E. Sexual dysfunction

267. Which of the following statements with regards to tricyclic antidepressants is least true?

    A. They are H_2 blockers.
    B. They have anticholinergic properties.
    C. They are adrenergic alpha$_1$ blockers.
    D. They are arrhythmogenic.
    E. They increase the seizure threshold.

268. Which one of the following is least likely to be an example of a G-protein receptor?

    A. Alpha$_1$
    B. Alpha$_2$
    C. D_1
    D. D_2
    E. $GABA_A$

269. Which of the following terms best describes the process where a section of a DNA molecule unzips and one of the DNA strands acts as a template for the synthesis of RNA?

    A. Adhesion
    B. Binary connection
    C. Transcription
    D. Triangulation
    E. Translation

264. Answer: E. PCR is a method to selectively amplify small regions of the genome up to 10 000-fold. This eliminates the need to perform a Southern blot analysis. It is a technique to amplify DNA resulting in numerous copies of a particular DNA sequence. The method relies on thermal cycling, consisting of cycles of repeated heating and cooling of the reaction for DNA melting and enzymatic replication of the DNA. Primers (short DNA fragments) containing sequences complementary to the target region along with a DNA polymerase (after which the method is named) are key components to enable selective and repeated amplification. As PCR progresses, the DNA generated is itself used as a template for replication, setting in motion a chain reaction in which the DNA template is exponentially amplified. PCR can be extensively modified to perform a wide array of genetic manipulations. (31, pp 158–9)

265. Answer: C. The five constructs that are integral to the psychoanalytic conception of the mind are dynamic, topographical, economic, structural and genetic. Most of the current psychoanalytic theories and practice are based on these five concepts. (31, pp 1770–1)

266. Answer: C. Selective serotonin reuptake inhibitors (SSRIs) like paroxetine appear to be an important peripheral mediator in the pain transmission of efferent pathways. They have been used in the management of pain syndromes such as peripheral neuropathy, chronic headaches and fibromyalgia. The common side effects of paroxetine are dry mouth, some weight gain, headaches, hyponatreamia and increased risk of gastrointestinal bleeds. (31, pp 2066–77)

267. Answer: E. Tricyclic antidepressants lower the seizure threshold. Caution is required with other proconvulsive drugs like antipsychotic medications, particularly if the patient is being treated for epilepsy. (32, p 247)

268. Answer: E. All the receptors important to psychiatry, with the exception of the ion channel glutamate and $GABA_A$ receptors, are G-protein receptors. (31, p 583)

269. Answer: C. Transcription is the synthesis of RNA under the direction of DNA. RNA synthesis, or transcription, is the process of transcribing DNA nucleotide sequence information into RNA sequence information. Both nucleic acid sequences use complementary language, and the information is simply transcribed, or copied, from one molecule to the other. DNA sequence is enzymatically copied by RNA polymerase to produce a complementary nucleotide RNA strand, called messenger RNA (mRNA), because it carries a genetic message from the DNA to the protein-synthesising machinery of the cell. (31, pp 37–8)

270. Which of the following best describes a brief transitional state between wakefulness and sleep, characterised by mixed frequency EEG and slow wave movements?

A. Sleep latency
B. Stage 1 sleep
C. Stage 2 sleep
D. Stage 3 sleep
E. Stage 4 sleep

271. In relation to autosomal dominant inheritance, which one of these statements is least likely to be true?

A. They arise from a mutation of the sex chromosomes.
B. Individuals have one (heterozygous) or two (homozygous) mutant genes.
C. Huntington's disease is an example.
D. They occur in half of all individuals in a sibship.
E. Most common in Mendelian disorders.

272. A 42-year-old man with bipolar disorder, treated with lithium carbonate 1000 mg for the past year, presents to Casualty with lethargy, weakness, fever and tremulousness. He is diagnosed with an encephalopathic syndrome. This disorder was attributed to another of his prescribed medications. Which of the following medications is most likely to cause this syndrome with lithium use?

A. Non-steroidal anti-inflammatory
B. Ferrous sulphate
C. Neuroleptic medication
D. Penicillin
E. Vitamin supplement

273. Which of the following is least likely to be true when it comes to describing someone with a dissocial personality disorder?

A. Callous unconcern for the feeling of others
B. Disregard for rules and obligations
C. Fear of abandonment
D. Inability to experience guilt
E. Tendency to blame others

274. A 25-year-old man who is a chronic heavy cigarette smoker with a diagnosis of schizophrenia was recently started on an antipsychotic medication for his illness. Which one of the following antipsychotic medications is most likely to be affected, given this man's level of smoking?

A. Risperidone
B. Clozapine
C. Quetiapine
D. Ziprasidone
E. Sertindole

270. Answer: C.

Stage 2 sleep is the state between wakefulness and sleep. In humans, each sleep cycle lasts from 90 to 110 minutes on average, and each stage may have a distinct physiological function. Stage 2 is characterised by sleep spindles ranging from 12 to 16 Hz and K-complexes. During this stage, muscular activity as measured by EMG decreases, and conscious awareness of the external environment disappears. This stage occupies 45–55% of total sleep in adults. (31, pp 80–1)

271. Answer: A.

Autosomal dominant diseases are uncommon. In the case of these diseases, the dominant gene causes a defect. Often such diseases cause death before a person can bear offspring. For that reason they are eliminated by evolutionary pressures. Autosomal dominant diseases that do not appear until after sexual maturity have a chance of being spread to offspring. This is the case in Huntington's disease. (30, pp 39–40)

272. Answer: C.

An encephalopathic syndrome characterised by weakness, lethargy, fever, tremulousness and confusion, extrapyramidal symptoms, leucocytosis, elevated serum enzymes, and elevated blood urea nitrogen has occurred in several patients treated with lithium plus a neuroleptic. In some cases, the syndrome was followed by irreversible brain damage. Due to the possible causal relationship between these events and the concomitant administration of lithium and neuroleptics, patients receiving such combined therapy should be monitored closely for early evidence of neurologic toxicity and treatment should be discontinued promptly if such signs appear. This encephalopathic syndrome may be similar to or the same as neuroleptic malignant syndrome (NMS). (33)

273. Answer: C.

Fear of abandonment is common in dependant personality disorder. Callous unconcern for others, disregard for rules and norms, inability to maintain enduring relationships, low frustration tolerance, incapacity to experience guilt and a marked proneness to blame others are ICD-10 diagnostic criteria for dissocial personality disorder. (34, pp 204–6)

274. Answer: B.

Clozapine and olanzapine are two antipsychotic medications that are substrates for cytochrome P4501A2, and cigarette smoking induces this enzyme system. Clozapine, quetiapine, ziprasidone and sertindole are substrates for cytochrome P4503A4 enzyme system. This system is not affected by cigarette smoking. Risperidone, clozapine and olanzapine are substrates for cytochrome P4502D6 enzyme system that is not affected by cigarette smoking. Risperidone's metabolite is also an active antipsychotic (9-OH-risperidone). (3, pp 437–40)

275. A 50-year-old woman with a diagnosis of bipolar disorder and epilepsy has been well maintained on sodium valproate. She recently had a relapse of both illnesses after a second medication was introduced. Which of these medication is mostly likely responsible for her relapse?

A. Carbamazepine
B. Lamotrigine
C. Clonazepam
D. Levetiracetam
E. Diazepam

276. A 30-year-old man with a diagnosis of treatment-resistant schizophrenia has been on high-dose clozapine medication. To reduce his risk of seizures, an anticonvulsant medication was introduced. He developed agranulocytosis requiring the intervention of a haematologist. Which of these anticonvulsant medications is most likely responsible for his agranulocytosis in combination with clozapine?

A. Sodium valproate
B. Lamotrigine
C. Carbamazepine
D. Clonazepam
E. Levetiracetam

277. A 30-year-old man with a diagnosis of schizoaffective disorder being treated with clozapine medication was found to have mild neutropenia on routine blood investigation. Which of these psychotropic medications is most likely to have a beneficial effect in correcting this man's neutropenia?

A. Olanzapine
B. Risperidone
C. Lamotrigine
D. Sodium valproate
E. Lithium carbonate

278. A 50-year-old man was recently diagnosed with bipolar affective disorder. He was stabilised on lithium carbonate. He later developed hypertension requiring antihypertensive medication. Which of these antihypertensive medications has the least potential for interaction with lithium?

A. Ramipril
B. Frusemide
C. Bendroflumethiazide
D. Losartan
E. Atenolol

275. Answer: A. Carbamazepine is an important cytochrome P450 liver enzyme inducer that could cause a decrease in the level of sodium valproate. A useful mnemonic used in remembering the common cytochrome P450 liver enzyme inducers is **PC-BRAS**. **P** – Phenytoin, **C** – Carbamazepine, **B** – Barbiturates, **R** – Rifampicin, **A** – Alcohol **(in chronic excess)**, **S** – Sulphonylureas. The important liver enzyme inhibitors are remembered by the mnemonic **ODEVICES**. **O** – Omeprazole, **D** – Disulfiram, **E** – Erythromycin, **V** – Valproate, **I** – Isoniazid, **C** – Cimetidine/Ciprofloxacin, **E** – Ethanol (in acute intoxication), **S** – Sulphonamides. SSRI antidepressants particularly fluoxetine, fluvoxamine, paroxetine and the antifungal medication ketoconazole are also important liver enzyme inhibitors. (35, p 66)

276. Answer: C. The combination of carbamazepine and clozapine may increase the risk of agranulocytosis. They are therefore best avoided in combination. Sodium valproate is recommended for prophylactic use in patients on clozapine in high doses or with plasma levels $> 500 \ \mu g/L$. (2, pp 71, 154)

277. Answer: E. Lithium carbonate has been found to be useful in increasing white blood cell count in patients who have developed neutropenia with clozapine. Olanzapine, risperidone, lamotrigine and sodium valproate may play a role in this patient's treatment; however there is no evidence to suggest that they increase white cell count. (36)

278. Answer: E. Thiazide diuretics, e.g., bendroflumethiazide; loop diuretics, e.g., frusemide; angiotensin-converting enzyme (ACE) inhibitors, e.g., ramipril; angiotensin II receptor antagonists, e.g., lorsatan; and non-steroidal anti-inflammatory drugs, e.g., ibuprofen, are well recognised in clinical practice to cause significant drug interaction with lithium, which may lead to lithium toxicity. Atenolol, a beta-1 receptor blocker, is not known to cause any significant interaction with lithium and may be a safer option in combination with lithium. (2, p 150)

279. A 60-year-old man with a long history of alcohol dependence syndrome was recently diagnosed with Wernicke's encephalopathy. Which of the following clinical features is the most common in patients with this condition?

    A. Liver disease
    B. Serious malnutrition
    C. Peripheral neuropathy
    D. Gait abnormalities (ataxia)
    E. Ocular abnormalities (nystagmus, sixth nerve palsy, conjugate gaze palsy)

280. A 35-year-old man with a diagnosis of schizophrenia presented with loss of libido and non-compliance with his antipsychotic medication, risperidone. This man's psychiatrist attributed his loss of libido to risperidone. Which of these options best explains the aetiology of loss of libido due to risperidone in this patient?

    A. Mesolimbic dopaminergic receptor antagonism
    B. Serotonergic (5HT2A) receptor antagonism
    C. Serotonergic (5HT7) receptor antagonism
    D. Alpha$_1$ receptor antagonism
    E. Alpha$_2$ receptor antagonism

281. A 24-year-old woman who is two weeks postpartum develops a sudden onset of a psychotic disorder with symptoms of elation, euphoria, rambling speech, flight of ideas, lability of mood, confusion and overactivity. From recent genetic evidence, which one of the following genes is most likely related to this psychiatric disorder?

    A. Neuregulin-1 (NRG-1), a susceptibility gene on chromosome 8p.
    B. Dysbindin (DTNBP1), a susceptibility gene on chromosome 6p.
    C. D-amino acid (*DAO*) and D-amino acid oxidase activator (DAO-A), a susceptibility gene identified within the chromosome 13q linkage region.
    D. Serotonin transporter gene, with linkage evidence pointing to the long arm of chromosome 16.
    E. Regulator of G protein signalling 4 (RGS-4) with linkage region on 1q.

282. In what proportion of deliveries does puerperal psychosis most likely occur?

    A. 1 in 10
    B. 1 in 100
    C. 1 in 200
    D. 1 in 1000
    E. 1 in 10 000

283. A monozygotic twin sibling of a patient with schizophrenia asks you, his brother's psychiatrist, what is his risk of developing schizophrenia. Which one of the following best estimates his lifetime risk of developing schizophrenia?

    A. 46%
    B. 48%
    C. 13%
    D. 17%
    E. 9%

279. Answer: E. All the options A–E are common in patients with Wernicke's encephalopathy; however, the most common are ocular abnormalities. They are present in about 96% of patients on initial examination. Ataxia was observed in about 87% of patients who were testable. Peripheral neuropathy was present in about 82% of cases and was usually confined to the lower limbs. Serious malnutrition was evident in about 84% while 66% of patients showed evidence of liver disease. (37, p 578)

280. Answer: A. The human sexual response has three stages. The first stage is libido (desire for sex) mediated by mesolimbic dopaminergic D_2 receptors resulting in hyperprolactinaemia (if D_2 receptors are blocked) that affects libido. The second stage is arousal mediated by nitrous oxide (NO) via cGMP and by acetylcholine receptors. The third stage is orgasm accompanied by ejaculation. Spinal serotonergic fibres inhibit orgasm via agonist action on 5HT2A while noradrenergic stimulation facilitates orgasm. Note that risperidone has antagonistic action on 5HT2A, 5HT7, D_2, alpha$_1$, and alpha$_2$ receptors. (3, pp 540–46)

281. Answer: D. The answer is post-partum psychosis. Eighty per cent of these patients present with prominent affective symptoms with mania or depression with psychotic symptoms. Neuregulin1, dysbindin, D amino acids activator (G72), regulator of G protein signalling (RGS-4) and COMT, a susceptibility gene on chromosome 22q, have been linked to both schizophrenia and bipolar affective disorder; however, ongoing molecular genetic studies of puerperal psychosis have shown interesting findings at the serotonin transporter gene (Coyle 2000) and linkage evidence pointing to the long arm of Chromosome 16 (Jones 2007). (38) (39, p 254)

282. Answer: D. Puerperal psychosis affects 1 in 500 to 1 in 1000 deliveries. The recurrence rates following subsequent pregnancies are 50% or more, and about 50% of women have further non-puerperal episodes (Robertson 2005). (38)

283. Answer: B. Lifetime schizophrenia risks for degrees of genetic relatedness to a patient with schizophrenia. (39, p 253 (Table 18.5 Gottesman 1991))

Relative	Lifetime risk of schizophrenia(%)	Degrees of genetic relatedness
Monozygotic twin sibling of patient	48	First
Child of patient, other parent with schizophrenia	46	First
Dizygotic twin sibling of patient	17	First
Sibling of patient, one of patient's parents has schizophrenia	17	First
Child of patient, other parent healthy	13	First
Sibling of patient	9	First

284. A patient presented with recurrent viral and fungal infection and tetany. His physical and laboratory investigations revealed cardiac defects, abnormal facies, thymic hypoplasia, cleft palate, hypocalcaemia and microdeletion of chromosome 22q. From which one of the following psychiatric disorders is this patient most likely suffering?

A. Depressive disorder
B. Bipolar affective disorder
C. Obsessive compulsive disorder
D. Anxiety disorder
E. Schizophrenia

285. A 50-year-old female monozygotic twin informed her psychiatric team that her co-twin has a diagnosis of depressive disorder. Which of the following is least correct regarding this woman's genetic aetiology?

A. Twin studies show a concordance rate in monozygotic twins of approximately 40–50%.
B. Twin studies show a concordance rates in dizygotic siblings of approximately 25%.
C. The heritability of unipolar depressive disorder is approximately 70%.
D. There is compelling evidence of a true Mendelian mode of inheritance.
E. Genetic polymorphism within variants of the serotonin transporter (5HTT) gene has been associated with mood disorder.

286. A 21-year-old woman who has a diagnosis of systemic lupus erythematosus (SLE) presented with delusions and hallucinations. The liaison psychiatrist made a diagnosis of neuropsychiatric SLE (NPSLE). Which of the following antipsychotic medications is best recommended for the treatment of NPSLE?

A. Chlorpromazine
B. Haloperidol
C. Risperidone
D. Olanzapine
E. Sulpiride

287. An infantry soldier was diagnosed with post-traumatic stress disorder (PTSD) following his retirement 12 years after he was involved in a life-threatening combat. He coped with his symptoms until his retirement. He attributed his ability to cope to 'group effect' in active military service. Which one of these is not 1 of the 11 curative factors, as described by Irvin D. Yalom, that may have helped this man to cope with his symptoms?

A. Instillation of hope
B. Universality
C. Altruism
D. Cohesiveness
E. Pairing

284. Answer: E.

This patient has a diagnosis of DiGeorge syndrome (velocardiofacial syndrome). The popular acronym is **CATCH 22**. **C** – Cardiac defects, **A** – Abnormal facies, **T** – Thymic hypoplasia, **C** – Cleft palate and microdeletion of chromosome 22. Twenty-five to thirty per cent of all people with this syndrome develop schizophrenia and 0.5% of people with schizophrenia have microdeletions in this region. Microdeletion in this region results in the loss of about 50-80 genes. This results in reduction in the gene encoding COMT, which has been identified also on chromosome 22. COMT acts by degrading catecholamines and has a role in cortical dopamine metabolism. Therefore, in the presence a compromised or low-activity COMT psychosis may result in this syndrome. These patients also have an elevated risk of intellectual disability. (40, p 82, 41)

285. Answer: D.

There is no compelling evidence of a true Mendelian mode of inheritance for unipolar depression. Recent evidence from linkage studies suggest a polygenic inheritance where several genes (e.g., in regions 15q, 17p and 8p) may contribute susceptibility to major depressive disorder. In addition, environmental factors interacting with genetic factors also play an important role in the aetiology of mood disorders. (39, pp 275–6, 42)

286. Answer: E.

Chlorpromazine is well known to cause drug-induced lupus. It may aggravate photosensitivity and complicate the existing manifestations of lupus First-generation antipsychotic medications, i.e. haloperidol, are not recommended because they may exacerbate neuropsychiatric SLE (NPSLE)-associated movement disorders. Stroke is one of NPSLE syndromes; therefore, risperidone and olanzapine should be avoided. Olanzapine and risperidone are known risk factors for cerebrovascular adverse events in elderly patients without SLE. Quetiapine and sulpiride are recommended as there are no reports of adverse effects in individuals with NPSLE. (43)

287. Answer: E.

Irvin D. Yalom (1968) described 11 curative factors that occur in a group. These are instillation of hope, universality, group cohesiveness, altruism, corrective recapitulation of primary family group, development of socialising techniques, imitative behaviour, catharsis (expression of pent-up feelings), existential factors, imparting information (education) and interpersonal learning. Pairing, dependency and fight/flight are the three basic assumptions according to W.R. Bion (1961). Bion focused on the unconscious defences of a group as a whole rather than the problems of individual group members. (44, pp 603–4)

288. An 18-year-old girl has presented numerous times to her local emergency department for treatment of deliberate self-harm symptoms. Which one of the following psychological interventions has been shown to have the strongest evidence in treating self-harming behaviour in adolescents?

A. Dialectical behaviour therapy (DBT)
B. Family therapy
C. Psychodynamic psychotherapy
D. Interpersonal therapy (IPT)
E. Multi-system therapy

289. Which one of the following psychological therapies is best avoided in patients with PTSD as it lacks sufficient evidence to support its use?

A. Trauma-focused cognitive behaviour therapy (TFCBT)
B. Eye movement desensitisation and reprocessing (EMDR)
C. Psychological debriefing
D. All of the above
E. None of the above

290. Interpersonal therapy (IPT) has been shown to be effective in the treatment of major depressive disorder and bulimia nervosa. IPT is closest associated with which one of the following?

A. Harry Stack Sullivan
B. Aaron Beck
C. Anthony Ryle
D. Marsha Linehan
E. Albert Ellis

291. A 50-year-old man who has a long-standing history of alcohol dependence syndrome asks his GP to prescribe disulfiram medication to help him address his alcohol dependence. Which of the following terms best describes this treatment?

A. Reciprocal inhibition
B. Aversion therapy
C. Compliance therapy
D. Response prevention
E. Biofeedback

288. Answer: A.

Dialectical behaviour therapy (DBT) is the only empirically supported treatment for adults with multiple mental health problems at risk of suicide. In a two-year randomised controlled trial, DBT reduced suicidal behaviour, inpatient days and anger ratings compared with treatment as usual. Family therapy, psychodynamic psychotherapy, interpersonal therapy and multisystem therapy do not have a sufficient evidence base in self-harming behaviour. (45)

289. Answer: C.

There is no evidence that single-session individual psychological debriefing is a useful treatment for the prevention of post-traumatic stress disorder after traumatic events. Trauma-focused CBT and EMDR have been shown to be of benefit in the treatment of PTSD. There is little evidence base for the effectiveness of other psychotherapies such as psychodynamic therapy. (44, pp 161–2, 46)

290. Answer: A.

IPT is based on the work of Harry Stack Sullivan (1953). IPT has two main aims: to reduce depressive symptoms and to address social and interpersonal problems associated with the onset of the symptoms. It is a structured, individual and time-limited (8–12 sessions) psychotherapy. CBT is the work of Aaron Beck. DBT is the work of Marsha Linehan. CAT is the work of Anthony Ryle. RET is the work of Albert Ellis. (47, pp 853–60)

291. Answer: B.

Aversion therapy: in this case the unpleasant negative stimulus, the effect of the disulfiram as it acts to prevent breakdown of ethanol in the body, is used to suppress unwanted drinking behaviour. Reciprocal inhibition: systematic desensitisation is coupled with a response that is incompatible with the anxiety, e.g., relaxation. Biofeedback: an individual uses information on an aspect of bodily function, e.g., blood pressure, to alter the function of that bodily function, usually in an indirect way such as relaxing. Response prevention: patient stops himself from performing a particular ritual despite having a strong urge to perform the ritual. Compliance therapy: methods used to improve patients compliance to treatment; psycho-education forms an important aspect of this therapy. (44, pp 522–23; 593–4)

292. In Erickson's stages of psychosexual development, which of the following statements is most correct?

A. There is a conflict of trust vs. mistrust between the ages of 0 and 18 months.
B. Autonomy is the main task between the ages of 0 and 18 months.
C. Crisis of integrity vs. despair occurs between 40 and 65 years.
D. Separation-individuation is part of Erickson's stages of psychosexual development.
E. Identity vs. role confusion occurs between the ages of 6 and 12 years.

293. Which one of the following is not a psychosocial vulnerability factor associated with depression according to George Brown's classic study of working class women?

A. Having three or more children under the age of 14 years
B. A lack of paid employment
C. A lack of a confidant
D. Poverty
E. Early maternal loss

294. A 25-year-old woman with a diagnosis of borderline personality disorder was recently admitted into a therapeutic community. Which of the following characteristics is most true regarding the treatment provided in the therapeutic community?

A. Presumed equality between all the staff and residents.
B. Consensus between all the staff members before a decision is taken.
C. Therapy carried out in large group settings.
D. Stratification of therapy between groups as it will be difficult to achieve uniformity.
E. Differences in standards adopted for individuals based on their cultural backgrounds.

295. According to Jean Piaget, if an equal amount of water is poured from a wide glass into a taller/thinner glass, a 4-year-old will pick the thinner and taller as containing more water. Which of the following best describes this stage of cognitive development?

A. Sensorimotor stage
B. Pre-operational stage
C. Concrete operational stage
D. Formal operational stage
E. None of the above

292. Answer: A.

Erickson described eight psycho-social stages of development (below). Separation-individuation is part of Margaret Mahler's objects relations theory. (48)

Stages	Age range	Basic conflict	Important event
1	0–18 months	Trust vs. mistrust	Feeding
2	18 months–3 years	Autonomy vs. shame and doubt	Toilet training
3	3–5 years	Initiative vs. guilt	Exploration
4	6–11 years	Industry vs. inferiority	School
5	12–18 years	Identity vs. role confusion	Social relationships
6	19–40 years	Intimacy vs. isolation	Relationships/Love
7	41–65 years	Generativity vs. stagnation	Work and parenthood
8	>65 years	Ego integrity vs. despair	Reflection on life

293. Answer: D.

Brown and Harris described four psychological vulnerability factors associated with the development of depression as described in the question. Poverty is not one of these factors; however poverty has been described as a risk factor for depression. (49, 50)

294. Answer: A.

Tom Main described therapeutic communities; an example is the Casell Hospital. The key principles include collective responsibility, citizenship and empowerment. Patients (called residents) with severe personality disorder are admitted and the regime is characterised according to Rapoport (1960) by 'permissiveness', 'reality confrontation', 'democracy' and 'communalism'. There is flattening of hierarchies, deliberate encouragement of personal responsibility and discouragement of unhelpful dependency on professionals – staff and residents are presumed to be equal. Differences between staff and residents are minimised and decisions are made with residents having a majority vote. (30, p 572)

295. Answer: B.

Jean Piaget, a Swiss biologist and developmental psychologist (1896–1980), identified four stages of cognitive development, A–D above. Sensorimotor stage (0–2 years): allows children to learn about their environment through sensory and motor systems, e.g., looking, feeding, touching and motor activity. The key achievement of this stage is object permanence; objects remain in exact position even when they are no longer in view. Preoperational stage (2–7 years): thinking in this stage is dominated by perception. This explains the action of this 4-year-old child; children at this stage pay attention to only part of a situation (centration). There is failure of conservation and reversibility. They think in an egocentric manner. Concrete operational (7–11/12 years): children become less dependent on perception and are able to achieve reversibility; however they are limited to concrete thinking and are inflexible in their thinking. Formal operational stage (11/12 years and above): children think in more abstract ways and are able to think in terms of possibilities rather than simply actual stages. (51, pp 111–6)

296. In relation to the epidemiology of bipolar affective disorder, which one of the following is least correct?

    A.   The prevalence of bipolar disorder as estimated by the epidemiological catchments area (ECA) study is 0.011.

    B.   The lifetime risk of bipolar disorder lies between 0.3% and 1.5%.

    C.   The prevalence in men and women is the same.

    D.   Female sufferers have proportionately fewer manic episodes.

    E.   The age of onset is later in bipolar disorder than in major depressive disorder.

297. In relation to the epidemiology of unipolar depression, which of the following is least correct?

    A.   The lifetime rate varies considerably in different studies; however, the true figure probably lies between 10% and 20%.

    B.   Before puberty, prevalence rates are similar in both sexes, but rise after puberty to about twice as great in women as in men.

    C.   The mean age of onset is about 27 years.

    D.   The 12-month prevalence of major depression in the community lies between 10% and 20%.

    E.   In the UK, the most common psychiatric diagnosis in people who have committed suicide is mood disorder.

298. In the report of the National Confidential Inquiries into Suicide and Homicide by People with Mental Illness (NCI 1999), which of the figures listed below best describes the percentage of people who were in contact with services within a week of their suicide?

    A.   9%

    B.   19%

    C.   29%

    D.   39%

    E.   49%

299. Which of the following antidepressants has the longest approximate half-life?

    A.   Citalopram

    B.   Escitalopram

    C.   Fluoxetine

    D.   Paroxetine

    E.   Sertraline

300. Which of the following is false with regard to sodium valproate?

    A.   It can cause hyperandrogenism in women.

    B.   Peak levels are lower if the 'chrono' form of the drug is used rather than the conventional form.

    C.   It can displace aspirin from albumin and cause aspirin toxicity.

    D.   Use may lead to hair loss with curly re-growth.

    E.   The anticonvulsant effects of sodium valproate are antagonised by antidepressant and antipsychotic medications.

296. Answer: E.

Community surveys in industrialised countries have suggested that the lifetime risk of bipolar disorder lies between 0.3% and 1.5%. Bipolar disorder has equal sex ratio, and an earlier age of onset compared with unipolar major depression. The mean age of onset is about 17 years for bipolar disorder compared with unipolar major depression, which is about 27 years. Female sufferers have proportionately fewer manic episodes. (44, pp 286–7)

297. Answer: D.

The 12-month prevalence of major depression in the community lies between 2% and 5%. Some other studies quote annual rates of 0.8% in Taiwan and 5.8% in New Zealand. (44, p 287, 47, pp 408–9)

298. Answer: E.

According to the National Confidential Inquiries into Suicide and Homicide by People with Mental Illness, 49% of the patients who died by suicide had been in contact with services in the previous week, while 19% had contact in the previous 24 hours. About 25% of all suicides had contact with mental health services in the year before their death. Sixteen per cent of this group were psychiatric inpatients at the time of death. According to the July 2010 publication of the NCI, the most common methods of suicide were hanging/strangulation, self-poisoning (overdose) and jumping/multiple injuries.

Suicide deaths by hanging and cutting/stabbing have increased, while death by self-poisoning, carbon monoxide (CO) poisoning, drowning and firearms have decreased. Figures for jumping and burning have remained stable. In males, the most common methods were hanging/strangulation, self-poisoning and jumping/multiple injuries. In females, self-poisoning was the most common method followed by hanging/strangulation. (52)

299. Answer: C.

All selective serotonin reuptake inhibitors (SSRIs) have long half-lives allowing once daily dosing. Approximate elimination half-lives of citalopram and escitalopram are 33 and 30 hours, respectively. The values for paroxetine and sertraline are 24 and 26 hours, respectively. Fluoxetine has an approximate half-life of 48-72 hours; however norfluoxetine, the active metabolite of fluoxetine, has an elimination half-life of 4-16 days. (2, pp 180–1)

300. Answer: C.

Sodium valproate is highly protein bound, but aspirin is more highly protein bound and can displace sodium valproate from albumin, thus leading to sodium valproate toxicity. Other less protein bound drugs such as warfarin can be displaced by sodium valproate. Many side effects of valproate are related to the peak plasma level. The 'chrono' form produces lower peak levels and may be better tolerated. (2, pp 144–5)

References

1. Craddock N, O'Donovan MC, Owen MJ. The genetics of schizophrenia and bipolar disorder: dissecting psychosis.
   J Med Genet. 2005; **42**(3):193–204.
2. Taylor D, Paton C, Kerwin R. *The South London and Maudsley NHS Foundation Trust Oxleas NHS Foundation Trust: prescribing guidelines*. 9th ed. London: Informa Healthcare; 2007.
3. Stahl S. *Essential Psychopharmacology, Neuroscientific Basis and Practical Applications*. 2nd ed. Cambridge: Cambridge University Press; 2000.
4. Hodges JR. *Cognitive Assessment for Clinicians*. Oxford; New York: Oxford University Press; 1994. xii, 242 pp.
5. Lishman WA. *Organic Psychiatry: the psychological consequences of cerebral disorder*. 3rd ed. Oxford; Malden, MA: Blackwell; 1988.
6. King D, editor. *Seminars in Clinical Psychopharmacology*. London: Royal College of Psychiatrists, Gaskell; 1999.
7. Puri B, Tyrer P. *Sciences Basic to Psychiatry*. Edinburgh; New York: Churchill Livingstone; 2000.
8. Anderson IM, Reid IC. *Fundamentals of Clinical Psychopharmacology*. London; New York: CRC Press; 2004.
9. National Collaborating Centre for Mental Health (UK). *Schizophrenia: core interventions in the treatment and management of schizophrenia in primary and secondary care (update)*. Leicester: British Psychological Society; 2009 March.
10. National Collaborating Centre for Nursing and Supportive Care (UK). *Violence: the short-term management of disturbed/violent behaviour in in-patient psychiatric settings and emergency departments*. London: Royal College of Nursing (UK); 2005 February.
11. Sadock BJ, Sadock VA, Kaplan HI. *Kaplan & Sadock's Comprehensive Textbook of Psychiatry*. 8th ed. Philadelphia, PA: Lippincott Williams & Wilkins; 2005.
12. Roth A, Fonagy P. *What Works for Whom?: a critical review of psychotherapy research*. New York: Guilford Press; 2004.
13. Afifi AK, Bergman RA. *Functional Neuroanatomy: text and atlas*. New York: Lange Medical Books/McGraw-Hill; 2005.
14. Puri BK, Hall AD. *Revision Notes in Psychiatry*. London: Arnold; 2004.
15. Crossman AR, Neary D. *Neuroanatomy: an illustrated colour text*. 2nd ed. Edinburgh; New York: Churchill Livingstone; 2000.
16. Hodges JR. *Cognitive Assessment for Clinicians*. Oxford; New York: Oxford University Press; 2005.
17. Buckley P, Bird J, Harrison G. *Examination Notes in Psychiatry: a postgraduate text*. Oxford; Boston, MA: Butterworth-Heinemann; 1998.
18. Gelder MG, López Ibor JJ, Andreasen NC. *New Oxford Textbook of Psychiatry*. Oxford: Oxford University Press; 2004.
19. Foley SR, Kelly BD, Clarke M *et al*. Incidence and clinical correlates of aggression and violence at presentation in patients with first episode psychosis. Schizophr Res. 2005; **72**(2-3):161–8.
20. Rösner S, Hackl-Herrwerth A, Leucht S *et al*. Opioid antagonists for alcohol dependence. Cochrane Database Syst Rev. 2010; **8**(12):CD001867.
21. Gillberg C. Deficits in attention, motor control, and perception: a brief review. Arch Dis Child. 2003; **88**(10):904–10.
22. Koro CE, Fedder DO, Gilbert JL *et al*. Assessment of independent effect of olanzapine and risperidone on risk of diabetes among patients with schizophrenia: population based nested case–control study. BMJ. 2002; **325**(7358):243.
23. Strachan P, Benoff B. Quetiapine overdose induced acute respiratory distress syndrome. Cest J. 2005; **128**(4_MeetingAbstracts):419S.
24. Agras WS, Walsh T, Fairburn CG *et al*. A multicenter comparison of cognitive-behavioral therapy and interpersonal psychotherapy for bulimia nervosa. Arch Gen Psychiatry. 2000; **57**(5):459–66.
25. Berryhill ME, Olson IR. The right parietal lobe is critical for visual working memory. Neuropsychologia. 2008; **46**(7):1767–74.
26. Dobkin BH. *The Clinical Science of Neurologic Rehabilitation*. New York: Oxford University Press; 2003.
27. Benes F. Neural circuitry models of schizophrenia: is it dopamine, GABA, glutamate, or something else? Biol Psychiatry. 2009; **65**(12):1003–5.
28. Rutter M, Taylor EA. *Child and Adolescent Psychiatry*. Oxford; Malden, MA: Blackwell; 2002.

29. Cormand B, Franke B. *The Role of Genetic Factors in Adult ADHD*. European College of Neuropsychopharmacology: Istanbul, Turkey; 2009. pp. 1–4.
30. Wright P, Stern J, Phelan M. *Core Psychiatry*. 2nd ed. Philadelphia, PA: Elsevier; 2005.
31. Kaplan HI, Sadock BJ. *Comprehensive Textbook of Psychiatry*. 6th ed. Baltimore, MD: Williams & Wilkins; 1995.
32. Taylor D, Paton C, Kerwin R. *Prescribing Guidelines*. 9th ed. London: Informa Healthcare; 2007.
33. Smith D, Keane P, Donovan J *et al*. Lithium encephalopathy. J R Soc Med. 2003; **96**(12):590–1.
34. World Health Organization. *The ICD-10 Classification of Mental and Behavioural Disorders: clinical descriptions and diagnostic guidelines*. Geneva: World Health Organization; 1992.
35. Kalra PA. *Essential Revision Notes for MRCP*. Revised ed. Cheshire: PasTest; 2002.
36. Blier P, Slater S, Measham T *et al*. Lithium and clozapine-induced neutropenia/agranulocytosis. Int Clin Psychopharmacol. 1998; **13**(3):137–40.
37. Lishman WA. *Organic Psychiatry: the psychological consequences of cerebral disorder*. 3rd ed. Oxford; Malden, MA: Blackwell; 1978.
38. Jones I, Smith S. Puerperal psychosis: identifying and caring for women at risk. Adv Psychiatr Treat. 2009; **15**(6):413–4.
39. Wright P, Stern J, Phelan M. *Core Psychiatry*. 2nd ed. Philadelphia, PA: Elsevier; 2005.
40. Schneider AS, Szanto PA. *Pathology*. Philadelphia, PA: Lippincott Williams & Wilkins; 2002.
41. Murphy KC, Owen MJ. Velo-cardio-facial syndrome: a model for understanding the genetics and pathogenesis of schizophrenia. Br J Psychiatry. 2001; **179**(5):397–402.
42. McGuffin P, Rijsdijk F, Andrew M *et al*. The heritability of bipolar affective disorder and the genetic relationship to unipolar depression. Arch Gen Psychiatry. 2003; **60**(5):497–502.
43. Mak A, Ho RCM, Lau CS. Clinical implications of neuropsychiatric systemic lupus erythematosus. Adv Psychiatr Treat. 2009; **15**(6):451–8.
44. Gelder M, Cowen P, Harrison P. *Shorter Oxford Textbook of Psychiatry*. Oxford; New York: Oxford University Press; 2006.
45. Wood A. Self-harm in adolescents. Adv Psychiatr Treat. 2009; **15**(6):434–41.
46. Rose SC, Bisson J, Churchill R *et al*. Psychological debriefing for preventing post traumatic stress disorder (PTSD). Cochrane Database Syst Rev. 2002;(2):CD000560.
47. Freeman CPL, Zealley AK. *Companion to Psychiatric Studies*. 6th ed. Johnstone EC, editor. Edinburgh: Churchill Livingstone; 1998.
48. Cherry K. Erik Erikson's Stages of Psychosocial Development, the eight stages of psychosocial development [accessed 14/03/2014]. Available from: http://psychology.about.com/od/psychosocialtheories/a/psychosocial.htm
49. Bruce ML, Takeuchi DT, Leaf PJ. Poverty and psychiatric status. Longitudinal evidence from the New Haven Epidemiologic Catchment Area study. Arch Gen Psychiatry. 1991; **48**(5):470–4.
50. Patten SB. Are the Brown and Harris 'vulnerability factors' risk factors for depression? J Psychiatry Neurosci. 1991; **16**(5):267.
51. Eysenck MW. *Simply Psychology*. 2nd ed. Hove; New York: Psychology Press; Taylor & Francis; 2002.
52. National Confidential Inquiry into Suicide and Homicide by People with Mental Illness. Manchester: The University of Manchester, 2010.
53. Korneva EA, Shanin SN, Rybakina EG. The role of interleukin-1 in stress-induced changes in immune system function. Neurosci Behav Physiol. 2001; **31**(4):431–7.

chapter 04

100 MCQs from Dr. Michael Reilly and Colleagues

Dr Mohamed Ali Ahmed; Dr Udumaga Ejike; Dr Ijaz Hussein; Dr Atif Ali Magbool; and Dr Gary McDonald

301. According to ICD-10, which of the following best describes the reliance on non-living objects as a stimulus for sexual arousal and sexual gratification?

A. Fetishism
B. Fetishistic transvestism
C. Frotteurism
D. Transsexualism
E. Voyeurism

302. Methadone is a licensed medication for heroin dependence treatment. Which of the following statements is most likely regarding methadone?

A. Appears to have a milder withdrawal syndrome than buprenorphine.
B. Is a controlled drug with a high dependency potential and a low lethal dose.
C. Is a long-acting opioid antagonist.
D. Is not recommended for women who are pregnant or planning a pregnancy compared with buprenorphine.
E. Should be prescribed in the oral tablet formulation.

303. Which of the following features best differentiates pseudo-dementia from dementia?

A. Affect is labile and shallow.
B. Attention and concentration are usually faulty.
C. Family are always aware of the dysfunction and its severity.
D. Patients conceal their disability.
E. Patients usually complain little of cognitive loss.

304. Regarding procedural memory, which of the following statements is least likely?

A. Basal ganglia, cerebellum and supplementary motor areas are involved.
B. It is a declarative.
C. It is explicit non-declarative.
D. It is implicit non-declarative.
E. The storage of memory last minutes to years.

301. Answer: A. Fetishistic transvestism is the wearing of clothes of the opposite sex principally to obtain sexual excitement. Frotteurism is rubbing up against people for sexual stimulation in crowded public places. Transsexualism is the desire to live and be accepted as a member of the opposite sex. Voyeurism is the persistent tendency to look at people engaging in sexual behaviour. (1, pp 215, 218–19)

302. Answer: B. Methadone should be prescribed in the liquid formulation, as tablets can be crushed and inappropriately injected. Buprenorphine appears to have a milder withdrawal syndrome than methadone. Methadone is a long-acting opioid agonist. Methadone is relatively safer than buprenorphine in women who are pregnant or planning a pregnancy. (2, pp 320–1)

303. Answer: C. Labile and shallow affect, faulty attention and concentration, concealment of disability and a lack of complaints relating to cognitive loss are all features of dementia. (3, p 339)

304. Answer: B. Procedural memory is explicit or implicit, non-declarative. Basal ganglia, cerebellum and supplementary motor area are involved. The storage of memory lasts minutes to years. (3, p 87)

305. A 24-year-old female recently diagnosed with a moderate depressive episode comes to your outpatient clinic worried about weight gain. What class of antidepressants is most likely to cause her weight gain?

A. Monoamine oxidase inhibitors
B. Noradrenaline reuptake inhibitors
C. Serotonin and noradrenaline reuptake inhibitors
D. Selective serotonin reuptake inhibitors
E. Tricyclic antidepressants

306. Which of the following antidepressant medications is most likely to cause significant postural hypotension?

A. Fluoxetine
B. Fluvoxamine
C. Lofepramine
D. Trazodone
E. Venlafaxine

307. Hyponatraemia is a potentially serious adverse effect of antidepressant medications. Which one of the following is least likely to be a risk factor for developing hyponatraemia?

A. Renal failure
B. Female sex
C. Increased body weight
D. Old age
E. Warm weather

308. One of the following drugs may decrease carbamazepine plasma concentration, and carbamazepine may increase or decrease its plasma concentration. Which of the following medications is the best fit to possess these properties?

A. Alprazolam
B. Clomipramine
C. Clozapine
D. Haloperidol
E. Phenytoin

309. A 21-year-old man with a family history of substance misuse attends his local addiction service asking the duty psychiatrist about his probability of becoming 'dependant on drugs'. If he has tried would he have at least once, which one he the highest probability of becoming dependent on?

A. Alcohol
B. Anxiolytics
C. Cannabis
D. Heroin
E. Tobacco

305. Answer: E. Tricyclic antidepressants (TCAs) as a group are potent antagonists of anti-histaminergic receptors. Anti-histaminic activity underlies the sedative side effects of TCAs. As a consequence of sedative properties, TCAs can increase somnolence. Anti-histaminic activity also contributes to the most unwanted adverse effect for patients, weight gain. Weight gain on TCAs can be considerable and is a factor for non-adherence. The likelihood is greatest with amitriptyline and least with the secondary amines. (4, p 273)

306. Answer: D. Trazodone can cause significant postural hypotension. Lofepramine causes a lesser degree of postural hypotension compared with other TCAs. Fluoxetine, fluvoxamine and paroxetine cause minimal effect on blood pressure. Venlafaxine at higher doses can cause hypertension. (2, p 224)

307. Answer: C. Most antidepressant medications have been associated with hyponatraemia, which is a serious adverse effect that needs careful monitoring, particularly in those patients at greatest risk, those i.e., of older age, female gender, low body weight, low baseline sodium concentration, reduced renal function and experiencing warm weather. (2, p 210)

308. Answer: E. Carbamazepine may decrease drug plasma concentration of alprazolam, amitriptyline, clomipramine, haloperidol, hormonal contraceptives, phenytoin and warfarin. It may increase drug plasma concentration of clomipramine, phenytoin and primidone. Drugs that may decrease carbamazepine plasma concentrations are cisplatin, phenobarbital, phenytoin and valproate. (3, p 1032)

309. Answer: E. Probability of becoming dependent when someone tried a substance at least once is tobacco 32%, heroin 23%, cocaine 17%, alcohol 15%, anxiolytics 9%, cannabis 9%, analgesics 8% and inhalants 4%. (5, p 968)

310. Which one of the following is least advisable on prescribing depot antipsychotic medication?

A. Adjust doses only after an adequate period of assessment
B. Administer at the shortest possible licensed interval
C. Begin with the lowest therapeutic dose
D. Give a test dose
E. None of the above

311. Regarding temperament, which of the following is most correct?

A. Antisocial personality disorder is associated with high levels of reward dependence.
B. Borderline personality disorder is associated with high levels of harm avoidance.
C. Histrionic personality disorder is associated with high levels of novelty seeking.
D. Passive-aggressive personality disorder is associated with low levels of novelty seeking.
E. Borderline personality disorder is associated with low levels of novelty seeking.

312. Regarding Freud dream theory, which one of the following terms best describes the latent content of the dream?

A. Actual content of the dream
B. Intellectual understanding of the dream by the dreamer
C. Masked meaning of the dream
D. Single image represents several unconscious wishes
E. Visual expression of hidden ideas

313. Regarding cognitive behaviour therapy, which of the following statements is least likely?

A. Mainly uses here and now rather than the past
B. Open and explicit
C. Sets behavioural tasks
D. Therapist is more active
E. Uses symbolism

314. In classical psychoanalysis the patient is typically asked to lie on a couch and to free-associate, saying whatever comes to mind without any type of censorship. The analyst sits behind the patient, remaining a relatively shadowy and neutral figure. Which of the following statements best describes the reasoning for this?

A. To be able to observe the patient better.
B. To encourage the development of transference.
C. To make the patient feel comfortable.
D. To maintain an appropriate level of communication.
E. To prevent the development of counter-transference.

310. Answer: B.

It is advisable on prescribing depot antipsychotic medication to administer at the longest possible licensed interval, give a test dose, begin with the lowest therapeutic dose and adjust doses only after an adequate period of assessment. There is no evidence to suggest that shortening the dose interval improves efficacy. (2, p 42)

311. Answer: B.

Borderline personality disorder is associated with high levels of harm avoidance. Novelty seeking, harm avoidance and reward dependence are temperament traits that influence personality. There is a significant genetic component to the heredity of temperament traits, with over 50% of the variance in traits being inherited. Different levels of these traits influence the person's risk of personality disorder, e.g., antisocial personality is associated with high novelty seeking, low harm avoidance and low reward dependence. (6, pp 2094–6)

312. Answer: C.

Manifest content is the actual content of the dream. Latent content is the masked meaning of the dream. Symbolism is visual expression of hidden ideas. Condensation is where a single image represents several unconscious wishes. Secondary revision is the intellectual understanding of the dream by the dreamer. (4, p 312)

313. Answer: E.

Cognitive behavioural therapy differs from other psychotherapies by being explicit and structured. It sets behavioural tasks, uses specific cognitive techniques and requires the therapist to be more active. (4, p 316)

314. Answer: B.

In classical psychoanalysis the analyst sits behind the patient, remaining a relatively shadowy and neutral figure to encourage the development of transference, because if the analyst becomes too human or real, then transference cannot develop easily. (7, p 465)

315. Regarding autosomal dominant transmission, which of the following is least likely?

    A. Females and males are affected.
    B. Male-to-male transmission does not take place.
    C. The phenotypic trait does not skip generations.
    D. Vertical transmission takes place.
    E. The phenotypic trait is present in all individuals carrying the dominant allele.

316. Which one of the following psychiatric illnesses has the strongest genetic effect?

    A. Alcohol dependence syndrome
    B. Anorexia nervosa
    C. Attention-deficit hyperkinetic disorder
    D. Bipolar disorder
    E. Schizophrenia

317. A 28-year-old pregnant woman is referred to your psychiatric outpatient clinic worried about her alcohol use during pregnancy. Which of the following regarding fetal alcohol syndrome is least likely?

    A. Occurs in one-third of all infants born to alcoholic women.
    B. Is characterised by delayed development, intellectual deficit and seizures.
    C. Is characterised by growth retardation of prenatal origin (height, weight).
    D. Is characterised by macrocephaly.
    E. Is characterised by microphthalmia.

318. Regarding causes of Down's syndrome, which of the following is most likely?

    A. Approximately 95% of cases result from trisomy 21 following non-disjunction during meiosis.
    B. Approximately 95% of cases result from trisomy 21 following non-disjunction during mitosis.
    C. Approximately 1% results from translocation involving chromosome 14.
    D. Approximately 1% results from translocation involving chromosome 21.
    E. Approximately 4% of cases are mosaics.

319. Which of the following statements best describes the epidemiology of bulimia nervosa?

    A. Ninety per cent of suffers are female.
    B. It tends to have an earlier age of onset compared to anorexia nervosa.
    C. The incidence in the UK has decreased.
    D. The incidence appears to be lowest in large cities.
    E. The incidence appears to be highest in rural areas.

320. Which of the following is most likely to be associated with stress-induced changes in the immune system of rodents?

    A. Decreased macrophage cytotoxic activity
    B. Decreased natural killer cell activity
    C. Diminished delayed-type hypersensitivity
    D. Decreased interferon production
    E. Leucopenia

315. Answer: B.

Autosomal dominant disorders result from the presence of an abnormal dominant allele causing the individual to manifest the abnormal phenotypic traits. The phenotypic trait is present in all individuals carrying the dominant allele and does not skip generations (vertical transmission takes place). Male and female are affected. Male-to-male transmission can take place. Transmission is not solely dependent on parental consanguineous mating. (8, pp 275–76)

316. Answer: C.

Association between a genetic risk factor and a disease in a population can be expressed as a relative risk. The relative risk of common psychiatric conditions derived from family studies are the following: attention-deficit hyperkinetic disorder = 55, autism = 45, schizophrenia = 10, bipolar disorder = 7, alcohol dependence = 6, generalised anxiety disorder = 2–5, anorexia nervosa = 2–4, unipolar depression = 1.5–3.0. (4, p 158)

317. Answer: D.

Fetal alcohol syndrome affects about one-third of all infants born to alcoholic women. The syndrome is characterised by growth retardation of prenatal origin (height, weight), minor anomalies, including microphthalmia, short palpebral fissure, midface hypoplasia, a smooth or short philtrum and a thin upper lip. Central nervous system manifestations include microcephaly, delayed development, hyperactivity, attention deficits, intellectual deficits and seizures. (3, p 20)

318. Answer: A.

The cause of Down's syndrome in approximately 95% of cases is trisomy 21. Another 4% is caused by translocation involving chromosome 21. The remaining cases are due to mosaics. (8, p 280)

319. Answer: A.

Bulimic symptoms are relatively common in the general population. Ninety per cent of sufferers are female. Bulimia nervosa tends to have a later age of onset, typically 18 year of age. In the UK, the incidence of cases presenting to primary care increased threefold between 1988 and 1993. The incidence seems to be highest in large cities, intermediate in urbanised areas and lowest in rural areas. (9, p 231)

320. Answer: D.

In the passive avoidance and learning task in mice, stress-induced changes cause decreased interferon production, delayed allograph rejection, decreased antibody response to challenge and increased death rate. Stress of different durations and intensities induced the formation of lymphocyte-activating factors by peritoneal macrophages and increased IL-1 α levels in mouse blood but led to different changes in the responses of target thymocytes to the committing actions of IL-1B that correlated with changes in the level of the humoral immune response. (10, pp 122–33, 11)

321. Which of the following is the most powerful predictor of suicide?

A. Adverse life events
B. Isolation
C. Male gender
D. Mental disorder
E. Unemployment

322. Which one of the following neuroimaging techniques is most likely to give information about regional cerebral blood flow, ligand binding and metabolic changes in the brain?

A. CT scan
B. MRI scan
C. PET scan
D. SPECT scan
E. X-ray

323. A 24-year-old male involved in a road traffic accident two years ago presents to your psychiatric outpatient clinic with a history of changes in his personality, disturbed mood, poor judgement, impaired motivation, social awareness and childishness. Which part of his brain is most likely affected?

A. Amygdala
B. Frontal lobe
C. Occipital lobe
D. Parietal lobe
E. Temporal lobe

324. Regarding resting membrane ion permeability, which of the following is most likely to be correct?

A. Chloride ions are freely permeable
B. Organic anions are relatively permeable
C. Potassium ions are relatively impermeable
D. Potassium ions are freely permeable
E. Sodium ions are relatively permeable

325. Which of the following is unlikely to be correct regarding macroscopic changes in Alzheimer's disease?

A. Global brain atrophy
B. Neuronal loss
C. Sulcal widening
D. The atrophy is usually most marked in the frontal and temporal lobes
E. Ventricular enlargement

321. Answer: D.

The Hierarchical Model of Suicide is divided into primary, secondary and tertiary risk factors. Primary factors are seen as powerful predictors of suicide and do not require the presence of secondary or tertiary factors to remain active, for example, mental disorders and health care. Secondary factors are concerned with adverse aspects of everyday life, e.g., isolation and loss. They are powerful in the presence of primary factors but are weak alone. Tertiary factors are mainly demographic, e.g., male gender, marital status. They have a very low predictive power in the absence of primary or secondary factors. (4, p 663)

322. Answer: C.

Both PET and SPECT can give information about ligand binding and regional cerebral blood flow, but PET can also give information about metabolic changes in the brain. (8, pp 208–9)

323. Answer: B.

Damage to the prefrontal cortex results in changes in personality that broadly fit into categories of disturbed mood, poor judgement, impaired social awareness, and motivation and perseveration of speech and movement. Childishness may be a feature, including making jokes and performing pranks (witzelsucht). Other features include perseveration, both of speech and movements; palilalia, or repetition of phrases and sentences; and decreased verbal fluency. Damage to the temporal lobe can result in amnesia, personality disturbances and visual field or sensory deficits depending on the location of the lesion. Lesions in the dominant occipital lobe results in alexia without agraphia, colour agnosia and visual object agnosia. Lesions in the non-dominant occipital lobe result in visuospatial agnosia, prosopagnosia, metamorphopsia and complex visual hallucinations. The parietal lobe is involved in attention, integration of information and appropriate connections of sensory input to actions. Damage to the amygdala can result in impaired emotional processing of stimuli, impaired emotional learning and deficits in emotional perception and expression. (9, pp 15–17, 22)

324. Answer: A.

The comparative permeability to different ions of the resting neuronal membrane is as follows: potassium ions are relatively permeable, sodium ions are relatively impermeable, chloride ions are freely permeable, organic anions are relatively impermeable. (8, p 211)

325. Answer: B.

The macroscopic changes in Alzheimer's disease include global brain atrophy, ventricular enlargement and sulcal widening. Histological changes include neuronal loss, shrinking of dendritic branching, reactive astrocytosis, neurofibrillary tangles and senile plaques. (8, p 193)

326. John has a diagnosis of bipolar affective disorder and he is on haloperidol depot injection every month. Two years later he develops movements in his mouth diagnosed as tardive dyskinesia. Which of the following option is least suitable for him?

A. Reduce the dose of his depot injection
B. Commence levodopa
C. Change depot injection to an atypical antipsychotic depot
D. Tetrabenazine
E. Sodium valproate

327. A patient newly diagnosed with schizophrenia has adherence issues with antipsychotic medication. Which of the following approaches would best support adherence to medication?

A. Avoid informing the patient about the side effects of the medication.
B. Using oral medication rather than depot injection.
C. Using paliperidone instead of chlorpromazine.
D. Using higher doses at the start of treatment in order that patient's body can become quickly accustomed to the medication.
E. Providing psycho-education to patient but not to his family.

328. A 61-year-old lorry driver presents with a four-month history for depression. Further assessment revealed history of ataxia, fatigue, flulike symptoms and rapid cognitive impairment. His pupils are normal and there is no evidence of rash. What is the most likely diagnosis?

A. Alzheimer's disease
B. Creutzfeldt–Jakob disease, new variant type
C. Creutzfeldt–Jakob disease, sporadic type
D. Lyme disease
E. Neurosyphilis

329. Andrew has schizophrenia and is currently on an antipsychotic medication. His psychiatrist wishes to keep the drug plasma concentration at optimum levels. Which of the following is least true in this case?

A. Addition of fluoxetine will increase plasma levels of antipsychotic medication.
B. Using cimetidine will increase plasma levels of antipsychotic medication.
C. Using carbamezapine will reduce levels of antipsychotic medication.
D. Using barbequed food will increase plasma levels of antipsychotic medication.
E. Smoking will reduce the plasma levels of antipsychotic medication.

330. A 78-year-old man presents to the psychiatric clinic with memory impairment and behavioural difficulties. You diagnose him with Alzheimer's disease. His daughter, who works as a nurse, asks you about the pharmacological options available for treating this condition. Which of the following options has the best evidence for the treatment of Alzheimer's disease?

A. Using donepezil as a disease-modifying agent.
B. Using galantamine as a disease-modifying agent.
C. Using an anti-oxidant as a symptomatic treatment.
D. Using an anti-inflammatory agent as a disease-modifying agent.
E. Using memantine as a disease-modifying agent.

326. Answer: B.

Tardive dyskinesia is a side effect of antipsychotic medications, particularly the conventional antipsychotic treatments. It is usually developed after years of treatment. The other associated factors are female gender and affective psychosis. The treatment options in tardive dyskinesia include using an atypical antipsychotic, stopping anticholinergic medication, tetrabenazine and reducing the dose of the offending antipsychotic, benzodiazepine, vitamin E and fish oil. The common medications to avoid in this condition are anticholinergics, e.g., procyclidine and dopamine antagonists such as levodopa and bromocriptine. (12, pp 92–9, 13, p 186)

327. Answer: C.

Using medication that has an easy dosing regimen will enhance adherence by patients with their medication. Paliperidone has a longer half-life and is usually administered once a day while chlorpromazine needs to be dispensed at a higher frequency. Other factors that can improve adherence are the following: (1) compliance therapy; (2) psycho-education to the family; (3) medication supervision; (4) providing clear advice and (5) referral to day-hospitals, day-centres or community psychiatric nurses. (13, pp 26–7)

328. Answer: C.

In Creutzfeldt–Jakob disease, sporadic type, peak age of onset is 50–70 years, there is rapid cognitive impairment and evidence of psychiatric symptoms early in one-third of cases. In Creutzfeldt–Jakob disease, new variant type, 30 years is the mean age of onset, duration of illness is longer than 14 months, cognitive impairment is late and two-thirds of cases present with psychiatric symptoms. (14, pp 406–7, 15, pp 518–19)

329. Answer: D.

Phenothiazines, tricyclic antidepressants, haloperidol, grapefruit juice and nefazodone are a few examples of cytochrome enzyme inhibitors, while smoking, barbecued food, rifampicin and phenytoin are a few of the examples of cytochrome enzyme inducers that increase the plasma levels of other medications metabolised by the liver. (13, p 58)

330. Answer: E.

There are three types of agents used in the treatment of Alzheimer's dementia: (1) the preventive approaches, e.g., antioxidant, anti-inflammatory and hormonal treatments; (2) disease-modifying agents, e.g., memantine, and there is some evidence for monoamine oxidase inhibitors and (3) symptomatic treatment, e.g., acetyl cholinesterase inhibitors such as donepezil, galantamine and rivastigmine. (13, pp 353–58)

331. A young man presents to Accident and Emergency following a road traffic accident with impaired comprehension, naming, reading and writing difficulties. He also shows semantic irrelevancies in his speech. Which of the following best describes his condition?

A. Transcortical sensory aphasia
B. Transcortical motor aphasia
C. Deep dysphasia
D. Conduction aphasia
E. Sensory aphasia

332. A 25-year-old man was involved in a road traffic accident, sustaining a head injury with frontal lobe damage. Which of the following is least likely to occur in frontal lobe damage?

A. Inability to plan
B. Difficulty with attention
C. Working memory deficits
D. Difficulties with facial recognition
E. Motor deficits

333. A woman presents to your clinic with her son, who has been diagnosed with an autistic spectrum disorder. She is concerned about attachment difficulties. Which of the followings is least correct about attachment?

A. Selective attachment develops within the first six months of an infant's life.
B. Attachment behaviour is associated more with affection than with seeking food.
C. Attachment behaviour displayed by an infant is highly correlated with subsequent development and behaviour.
D. Secure attachment behaviour is related to child temperament.
E. Insecure attachment behaviour includes the inability to express affection in a comfortable way with the attachment figure.

334. A married couple were involved in a road traffic accident three months ago. They were referred to you by their general practitioner for psycho-education related to post-traumatic stress disorder (PTSD). From your knowledge of the epidemiology of PTSD, which of the followings is most true?

A. The husband's chance of developing PTSD is twice that of his wife.
B. The husband is four times more susceptible to develop symptoms of PTSD compared to his wife.
C. His wife's chances of developing PTSD are twice those of her husband.
D. They both have equal chances of developing PTSD.
E. The wife is four times more susceptible to developing symptoms of PTSD.

331. Answer: A. Transcortical motor aphasia is characterised by transient mutism and telegrammatic dysprosodic speech. Deep dysphasia presents with word repetition deficits and paraphasia. Conduction aphasia presents with naming deficits and impaired ability to repeat non-meaningful single words and word strings. Sensory aphasia presents with general comprehension deficits, neologisms and word retrieval deficits. (16, p 96)

332. Answer: D. Frontal lobe damage can lead to motor and cognitive symptoms that may not occur in every case. Cognitive symptoms include inability to plan, difficulties in attention and working memory disturbances. Facial recognition is a function of the parietal lobe and the lack of it is prosopagnosia. (16, p 98)

333. Answer: A. The infant develops selective attention after six months of age. (16, pp 128–30)

334. Answer: C. The risk of developing PTSD after traumatic events is 8–13% for men and 20–30% for women. Lifetime prevalence is estimated at 7.8% with almost double the chance in females. (17, p 368)

335. A young man presented with symptoms of psychosis and was commenced on atypical antipsychotic medication. His mother is concerned about the association between weight gain and atypical antipsychotics. Which of the following is least likely a proposed mechanism of weight gain caused by atypical antipsychotics?

    A. Atypical antipsychotics can slow rates of metabolism.
    B. Atypical antipsychotics increase prolactin levels.
    C. Atypical antipsychotics alter cortisol and insulin secretion.
    D. Atypical antipsychotics cause sedation resulting in reduced activity.
    E. Atypical antipsychotics stimulate the sympathetic ganglion.

336. A 78-year-old lady was referred by her general practitioner with symptoms of insomnia for the past two months. Which of the following is most true about the epidemiology of insomnia?

    A. It is prevalent in approximately 5% of the general population.
    B. It is more common in males.
    C. It is more common in middle age versus old age.
    D. Only 6% have clinically significant insomnia.
    E. It can be caused by antidepressant medication.

337. A 33-year-old man was referred to the psychiatric services by his GP with memory loss, a movement disorder and tics. Family history revealed that his father had a similar problem and was diagnosed with Huntington's disease. Which of the following is most true about this condition?

    A. It is an autosomal dominant disorder.
    B. It is an autosomal recessive disorder.
    C. It is an X-linked recessive disorder.
    D. It is an X-linked dominant disorder.
    E. There is no genetic defect in Huntington's disease.

338. A 16-year-old boy is brought to the psychiatric outpatients by his mother because of behavioural difficulties. His mother informs you that his behaviour is repetitive and that he is shy and has a limited social circle. On examination, you note the boy has large ears, large testicles and there is a murmur audible on auscultation in the mitral valve area. What is the most likely diagnosis?

    A. ADHD
    B. Autistic spectrum disorder
    C. Lesch–Nyhan syndrome
    D. Fragile X syndrome
    E. Hunter syndrome

339. A lesion in which of the following areas of the brain would most likely lead to loss of appetite?

    A. Amygdala
    B. Caudate nucleus
    C. Nucleus accumbens
    D. Lateral nucleus of hypothalamus
    E. Medial nucleus of hypothalamus

335. Answer: E. Another proposed mechanism is increased thirst with increased fluid intake and fluid retention. Factors that increase the risk of weight gain are female sex, previous pattern of overeating, narcissistic traits and family or personal history of obesity. (17, p 852)

336. Answer: D. Insomnia is a common problem; it is more common in females and in the elderly. It is prevalent in 30% of the general population but only 6% of people suffer clinically significant insomnia. Antidepressant medication, anti-parkinsonian medications, bronchodilators, and chemotherapy can all cause insomnia in the general population. (17, pp 392–3)

337. Answer: A. Huntington's disease is an autosomal dominant disorder with atypical repeat of CAG on chromosome 4. It usually starts in the early 30s and 40s with fatal results and the patient dying within 10–12 years. Patients present frequently with symptoms of anxiety and depression, but psychotic presentations also occur. There is no treatment for the disease, but symptomatic treatment can be provided. (17, p 172)

338. Answer: D. Fragile X syndrome is the most commonly inherited cause of learning disability. The syndrome is associated with a sequence of triplet repeats (CGG) at a site on the X chromosome. Lesch–Nyhan syndrome is a rare X-linked recessive condition, while Hunter syndrome is caused by iduronate sulphatase deficiency. (17, pp 708–9)

339. Answer: D. The amygdala, nucleus accumbens and caudate nucleus are part of the basal ganglia. These parts are associated with motor activity and emotional regulation. The hypothalamus is the centre for the autonomic motor system controlling appetite, rage, temperature, blood pressure and sexual function. Lesions of the upper lateral nucleus result in destruction of the hunger centre causing loss of appetite. Ventral-medial area lesions result in destruction of the satiety centre causing increased appetite. (18, pp 76–8)

340. A 42-year-old patient presented to Accident and Emergency with psychotic symptoms. His medical records show that he has Huntington's disease. His brain scan is most likely to show which of the following?

A. Diminished volume of the caudate nucleus
B. Increased volume of the substantia nigra
C. Reduced grey matter volume of the prefrontal cortex
D. Reduced grey matter volume of the sub-thalamic nucleus
E. Reduced white matter of the cerebellum

341. A 22-year-old man presented to your psychiatric outpatient clinic with hallucinations and delusions. He admits to recently using ketamine. Which of the following is the most likely proposed mechanism of his psychotic presentation?

A. Activation of metabotropic glutamate receptors
B. Blockade of kainite glutamate receptors
C. Blockade of NMDA receptors
D. Blockade of AMPA receptors
E. Activation of AMPA receptors

342. A 22-year-old woman presented with symptoms suggestive of emotionally unstable personality disorder. You want to assess her personality with a Minnesota Multiphasic Personality Inventory (MMPI). Which of the following is not a scale of the MMPI?

A. Hypochondriasis
B. Masculinity-femininity
C. Bipolar affective scale
D. Schizophrenia
E. Paranoia

343. A 25-year-old man is admitted to hospital with deliberate self-harm. He is illiterate. Which of the following tests is best suited to assess his personality?

A. Minnesota Multiphasic Personality Inventory
B. Rorschach inkblot test
C. California Personality Inventory
D. Eysenck Personality Questionnaire
E. Adjective checklist

344. A 32-year-old woman is diagnosed with a mild depressive episode. She is considered for cognitive behaviour therapy. Which of the following would be least likely to occur in a cognitive behaviour therapy session?

A. Graded assignment
B. Psycho-education
C. Distraction
D. Active interpretation
E. Thought rehearsal

340. Answer: A. Caudate nucleus volume is reduced in Huntington's disease. Substantia nigra volume reduction is noted in Parkinson's disease. Cerebellum lesions lead to cerebellar ataxia characterised by intention tremors. (18, pp 75–6)

341. Answer: C. Glutamate (glutamic acid) is an excitatory receptor. Its activation results in blockade and regulatory effects on dopamine in the basal ganglia. There are four types of glutamate receptors: NMDA, AMPA, kainite and metabotropic. Only NMDA receptor blockade results in a psychotic presentation. (18, p 104)

342. Answer: C. The MMPI is a self-reported questionnaire. Other scales on this inventory are lie, infrequency, suppressor, depression, hysteria, psychopathic deviance, psychasthenia, hypomania, social introversion, repression and ego strength. (18, pp 180–2)

343. Answer: B. Rorschach developed this projective personality test, which composed of ten inkblots serving as a stimulus for association. Five of the inkblots are black and white while other five include colours. Patients are shown those cards and their responses are interpreted. The other projective test is the Thematic Apperception Test. (18, pp 182–4)

344. Answer: D. CBT was developed by Aaron Beck in the 1960s. The techniques include cognitive and behaviour components. Behavioural components are activity scheduling, graded assignment, exposure and response prevention, distraction and relaxation. Cognitive techniques are psycho-education, identifying and challenging negative automatic thoughts, and keeping a diary of thoughts. (18, p 786)

345. Which of the following techniques would be most likely to occur in group therapy sessions?

    A. Mirroring
    B. Examination of parapraxes
    C. Flooding
    D. Traps
    E. Snags

346. In an 80-year-old man with Alzheimer's disease, which of the following histopathological changes is least likely to be seen in the temporal lobe?

    A. Granulovacuolar degeneration
    B. Hirano bodies
    C. Pick's bodies
    D. Neurofibrillary tangles
    E. Senile plaques

347. In a 45-year-old man with Huntington's disease, which one of the following macroscopic neuropathological changes is least likely to be seen?

    A. Marked atrophy of the corpus striatum
    B. Dilatation of the lateral ventricles
    C. Dilatation of the third ventricle
    D. Depigmentation of the substantia nigra
    E. Marked atrophy of the frontal lobe

348. Which of the followings is least likely to be a feature of rapid eye movement (REM) sleep?

    A. Increased heart rate
    B. Increased systolic blood pressure
    C. Increased respiratory rate
    D. Increased muscle tone
    E. Increased cerebral blood flow

349. A 25-year-old male construction worker presented to Accident and Emergency several days after a left-sided head injury at work with associated speech difficulties including poor articulation and sparse speech. Which of the following brain areas is most likely affected in this case?

    A. Superior temporal gyrus
    B. Posterior inferolateral region
    C. Frontal operculum
    D. Medial temporal region
    E. Inferior parietal lobules

345. Answer: A.   Mirroring is a group-specific process that means duplication of the experience. Another technique in group therapy is amplification whereby the intensity of an emotional experience is increased by sharing it in the group. Depending on the type of group involved, various cognitive or analytic techniques can be used in therapy. (17, pp 780–1)

346. Answer: C.   In Alzheimer's disease the histopathological changes in the cerebral cortex include neuronal loss, shrinking of dendritic branching, reactive astrocytosis, neurofibrillary tangles and senile plaques, while the histopathological changes seen commonly in the hippocampus (part of the temporal lobe) include granulovacuolar degeneration, Hirano bodies, neurofibrillary tangles and senile plaques. Pick's bodies on the other hand are seen in Pick's disease. (19, p 124)

347. Answer: D.   Depigmentation of the substantia nigra is a macroscopic change seen in idiopathic Parkinson's disease. All the other options in the question are part of the macroscopic neuropathological changes seen in Huntington's disease. (19, pp 131–2)

348. Answer: D.   During REM sleep there is a maximal loss of muscle tone. REM sleep is associated with increased sympathetic nervous system activation that will subsequently increase the rate of all physiological functions including heart rate, blood pressure, respiratory rate, cerebral blood flow and protein synthesis. (19, p 143)

349. Answer: C.   The frontal operculum consists of the Broca'a area. Lesions in this area can lead to expressive (motor aphasia) Broca's nonfluent aphasia. Superior temporal gyrus consists of Wernicke's area and lesions in this region can lead to receptive (sensory aphasia) Wernicke's fluent aphasia. Lesions in the posterior inferolateral region can lead to prosopagnosia and impaired object recognition. Left-sided lesions affecting the medial temporal region can lead to anterograde amnesia affecting verbal information. Left-sided lesions in the inferior parietal lobule can lead to conduction aphasia and tactile agnosia. (19, pp 109–10)

350. A 70-year-old woman diagnosed with Gerstmann's syndrome is least likely to present with which of the following features?

A. Agraphia
B. Dyscalculia
C. Finger agnosia
D. Right–left disorientation
E. Anosognosia

351. Structural neuroimaging has the least utility in which of the following clinical indications?

A. Intracranial expanding lesions
B. Demyelination changes
C. Cerebral infarction
D. Cerebral oedema
E. Cerebral blood flow

352. The mutation that changes the DNA codon but does not affect the produced amino acid is best described as which of the following?

A. Somatic mutation
B. Germinal mutation
C. Silent mutation
D. Nonsense mutation
E. Chromosomal mutation

353. In a 40-year-old man with Huntington's disease, the pattern of inheritance of this disease is best described as which of the following?

A. Autosomal recessive inheritance
B. Autosomal dominant inheritance
C. X-linked inheritance
D. Non-Mendelian inheritance
E. Chromosomal abnormalities

354. Which of the following lifetime risks of developing schizophrenia in relatives of a patient with schizophrenia is least likely?

A. General population: 1
B. Nephew/niece of a patient: 4
C. Dizygotic twin sibling of a patient: 35
D. Monozygotic twin sibling of a patient: 48
E. Parent of a patient: 6

350. Answer: E.

Gerstmann's syndrome is a disorder affecting the dominant parietal lobe and it consists of dyscalculia, right–left disorientation, finger agnosia and agraphia. Anosognosia is a disorder most likely associated with lesions affecting the non-dominant parietal lobe. (9, p 19)

351. Answer: E.

The structural CT and MRI scans are widely used in neuropsychiatric research. Their clinical uses include the detection of intracranial expanding lesions, shifts of intracranial structures, cerebral infarction, cerebral oedema, atrophy of brain structures and demyelination changes. On the other hand, applications relating to cerebral blood flow are best visualised using functional neuroimaging technologies including PET, SPECT and fMRI scanning. (19, pp 137–8)

352. Answer: C.

The silent mutation is a point mutation that changes the DNA codon but does not affect the amino acid inserted into the protein, while the nonsense mutation occurs where the sequence is changed to that of a stop codon, causing production of an incomplete protein. The mutation during mitotic division in cells that do not give rise to gametes is called a somatic mutation, while mutations in cell precursors of gametes are called germinal mutations. Chromosomal mutations involve a change in the number of chromosomes or rearrangement of sequences during DNA replication. (20, p 50)

353. Answer: B.

In autosomal dominant inheritance the disease gene is dominant; the phenotype is evident in both the heterozygotes and homozygotes. The affected/unaffected ratio for offspring is 1:1 and the disorder does not escape generations. Huntington's disease is a good example of this pattern of inheritance. Options A, B and C are considered the three major patterns of Mendelian inheritance. (9, p 50)

354. Answer: C.

The risk of schizophrenia is greatest when there are close relatives affected, several relatives affected, and when a monozygotic sibling is affected. The lifetime risk of schizophrenia in a dizygotic twin sibling of a patient is approximately 17 not 35. (9, pp 274–75)

355. Which of the following questionnaire response types closest reflects where the subject always tends either to agree or disagree with questions?

    A. Social acceptability
    B. Response set
    C. Bias towards centre
    D. Halo effect
    E. Hawthorne effect

356. Which of the following circumstances is least likely to increase the rate of absorption of drugs administered intramuscularly?

    A. Lipid-soluble drugs
    B. Drugs with low molecular mass
    C. Physical exercise
    D. Cardiac failure
    E. Emotional excitement

357. Which of the following is more suggestive of unipolar depression than bipolar depression?

    A. Later age of onset
    B. Hypersomnia and psychomotor retardation
    C. Psychotic features
    D. Early age of onset
    E. High frequency of depressive episodes

358. Which of the following is the most common reaction involved in the hepatic phase I metabolism of psychotropic drugs?

    A. Hydrolysis
    B. Oxidation
    C. Conjugation
    D. Reduction
    E. None of the above

359. In a 29-year-old male with schizophrenia on typical antipsychotic medication, which of the following side effects is most likely secondary to antidopaminergic action on the tuberoinfundibular pathway?

    A. Parkinsonism
    B. Pyrexia
    C. Dry mouth
    D. Low sperm count
    E. Urinary retention

355. Answer: B. Social acceptability is when the subject chooses the acceptable answer rather than the true one. Bias towards the centre occurs when the subject tends to choose the middle response and shun extremes. The Halo effect occurs when the answers are chosen to fit with previously chosen answers and the Hawthorne effect occurs when the subject improves an aspect of their behaviour simply in response to the fact that they are in an experiment. (21, p 5)

356. Answer: D. The rate of absorption of drugs administered intramuscularly is increased when the drugs are of low relative molecular mass or are lipid soluble. Increased muscle blood flow (e.g., with physical exercise or emotional excitement) also increases the rate of absorption intramuscularly. Cardiac failure reduces muscle blood flow and subsequently reduces the rate of absorption intramuscularly. (19, p 161)

357. Answer: A. Late age of onset is suggestive of unipolar depression. Bipolar depression is associated with atypical features of depression, including hypersomnia, psychomotor retardation, psychotic features, early age of onset and high frequency of depressive episodes. (22)

358. Answer: B. Hepatic phase I metabolism involves oxidation hydrolysis and reduction. Oxidation is the most common metabolic reaction. Conjugation is the main process in hepatic phase II metabolism. (19, p 164)

359. Answer: D. Antipsychotic medications antidopaminergic action on the tuberoinfundibular pathway causing hyperprolactinaemia may lead to galactorrhoea and menstrual disturbances in females and low sperm count and gynaecomastia in males. Pyrexia may result from the central antimuscarinic action, while dry mouth and urinary retention are secondary to peripheral antimuscarinic effects of antipsychotic medication. Parkinsonism is secondary to antidopaminergic action on the nigrostriatal pathway causing extrapyramidal symptoms. (19, p 166)

360. In the psychopharmacogenetics of schizophrenia, which of the following is most true?

A. Acute akathesia with antipsychotic medication has been associated with polymorphism of DRD3 and DRD2.
B. Polymorphism of DRD3 and DRD2 has been associated with antipsychotic-induced hyperprolactinaemia.
C. Resistance to antipsychotic medication is well documented in patients with CY2D6.
D. Weight gain with antipsychotic medication has been associated with polymorphism of DRD3 and DRD2.
E. Heat shock protein 30-1 in clozapine-induced agranulocytosis is well documented.

361. In a 23-year-old, single unemployed woman with borderline personality disorder who has a significant history of childhood emotional difficulties, which of the following phases of human development has been mostly affected in her early life to develop this condition?

A. Rapprochement sub-phase
B. Object constancy
C. Practicing sub-phase
D. Differentiation sub-phase
E. None of the above

362. In which of the following scenarios is lithium least likely to be effective?

A. Treatment of mania
B. Prophylaxis for bipolar disorder
C. Prophylaxis for unipolar disorder
D. Maintenance therapy for bipolar disorder
E. Augmentation in treatment-resistant depression

363. A 23-year-old woman who has obsessive-compulsive disorder (OCD) attended her psychiatric outpatient appointment with you. She revealed to you that she had a throat infection in the past with complications. Which is of the following is most true in OCD?

A. No genetic causality has been reported.
B. No association between streptococcal infection and OCD.
C. Life time prevalence of 20%.
D. Decreased activity in frontal lobe, basal ganglia and the cingulum has been demonstrated in PET studies.
E. Sleep EEG shows decreased rapid eye movement latency.

364. In assessing intelligence, which of the followings is least likely to be part of the verbal component of the Wechsler Adult Intelligence Scale (WAIS-III)?

A. Arithmetic
B. Information
C. Letter number sequencing
D. Digit span
E. Digit symbol

360. Answer: A. A polymorphism of DRD3 and DRD2 has been documented in antipsychotic-induced acute akathisia. In antipsychotic-induced hyperprolactinaemia, DRD2 Taq1A polymorphism has been associated. Heat-shock protein 70-1 and 70-2 variants have been implicated in clozapine-induced agranulocytosis. (23)

361. Answer: A. Separation individuation phase extends from 6 to 36 months of age. This phase of human development involves the infant's psychological birth as a separate person apart from the mother. Borderline personality disorder has been attributed to the lack of optimal maternal emotional availability during the rapprochement sub-phase (16-24 months) of separation individuation phase according to Kernberg (1979). (24, pp 593, 1747, 2927)

362. Answer: C. Lithium is not recommended as first-line drug in prophylaxis of unipolar disorder. It is used as a treatment of mania, prophylaxis for bipolar disorder, maintenance therapy in bipolar disorder and in augmentation in cases of treatment-resistant depression. (21, p 57)

363. Answer: E. Sleep EEG abnormality in OCD patients is comparable with those that have depression. Streptococcal infection has been associated with OCD. PET studies have demonstrated increased activity in the frontal lobe, basal ganglia and the cingulum. (25, p 14)

364. Answer: E. Wechsler Adult Intelligence Scale (WAIS-III) has two scales – verbal and performance with seven tests each. The verbal scale includes arithmetic, comprehension, digit span, information, letter number sequencing, similarities and vocabulary. The performance scale includes block design, digit symbol, matrix reasoning, object assembly, picture arrangement, picture completion and symbol search. (14, p 97)

365. A 19-year old man was recently diagnosed with paranoid schizophrenia. The risk of this man attempting suicide is best described by which of the following percentages?

A. 1%
B. 5%
C. 15%
D. 50%
E. 80%

366. Which of the following assessment tools would be least suitable for studying psychiatric morbidity in a large population?

A. General Health Questionnaire
B. Diagnostic Interview Schedule
C. Present State Examination
D. Quality of Life Interview
E. Minnesota Multiphasic Personality Inventory

367. A 20-year-old ballet dancer presents to you with symptoms suggestive of a depressive episode. She is agreeable to start antidepressant medication. Which of the following antidepressants is most likely to cause weight loss in this woman?

A. Sertraline
B. Fluoxetine
C. Citalopram
D. Amitriptyline
E. Clomipramine

368. Which one of the followings is least likely be part of the limbic lobe?

A. Septal nucleus
B. Cingulate gyrus
C. Parahippocampal gyrus
D. Subcallosal gyrus
E. Caudate nucleus

369. Which of the following assessment tools is self-rated?

A. Beck Depression Inventory
B. Psychiatric Assessment Schedules for Adults with Developmental Disabilities
C. Yale–Brown Scale
D. Scale for Assessment of Negative Symptoms
E. Edinburgh Postnatal Depression Scale

370. Which of the following is less likely to be associated with increased risk of suicide?

A. Unemployment
B. Physical illness
C. Alcoholism
D. Religious affiliation
E. Prison inmates

365. Answer: C. Suicide is the most common cause of premature death in schizophrenia. It accounts for 10–38% of all deaths. (17, p 190)

366. Answer: C. Present State Examination is a clinician-administered semi-structured clinical interview yielding clinical diagnosis. The other assessment tools are either self-report or non-clinician-administered structured interviews and are preferred for larger sample sizes. (17, pp 176—77)

367. Answer: B. While fluoxetine is associated with weight loss, paroxetine and fluvoxamine are known to cause slight weight loss. Sertraline has been noticed to cause limited weight gain while citalopram has no effect on weight. Tricyclic antidepressants are all associated with some weight gain. (17, p 853)

368. Answer: E. The caudate nucleus is part of the corpus striatum, which is one of the components of the basal ganglia. The limbic lobe is composed of cortical areas including the cingulate gyrus, parahippocampal gyrus, subcallosal gyrus, and amygdaloidal and septal nuclei. (19, pp 111–12)

369. Answer: A. The Yale–Brown Scale is used for obsessive-compulsive symptoms while Scale for Assessment of Negative Symptoms is used to assess negative symptoms of schizophrenia. Similarly Psychiatric Assessment Schedules for Adults with Developmental Disabilities is used as a screening tool for assessing psychiatric disorders in a learning-disabled population. The Edinburgh Postnatal Depression Scale is used for assessing symptoms of postnatal depression. The Beck Depression Inventory (BDI) is a self-rated questionnaire for depressive symptom screening. (3, p 298)

370. Answer: D. Religious affiliation is a protective factor against suicide. On the other hand, alcoholism, psychiatric morbidity, personality disorder, physical illness and being a prison inmate are all associated with increased rates of suicide. (21, pp 150–2)

371. A 50-year-old patient with schizophrenia living in a supported hostel is brought to the Accident and Emergency Department by a nurse from the hostel. He had been well until recently. He is complaining of headache and blurred vision, and is reported to have vomited twice that morning. On mental state examination, he describes persecutory paranoid beliefs but is fully orientated. Nursing staff note that he is more thirsty in the past few weeks. His blood glucose is normal. What other biochemical marker is most likely to be abnormal?

A. Bicarbonate
B. Chloride
C. Potassium
D. Sodium
E. Urea

372. A patient with schizophrenia who has good symptom control for several years on thioridazine develops abnormal movements, including lip-smacking and tongue protrusion. Changing to which medication is most likely to result in an improvement in these symptoms?

A. Aripiprazole
B. Clozapine
C. Olanzapine
D. Quetiapine
E. Risperidone

373. A 30-year-old man whom you commenced on amitriptyline four months ago has reported experiencing problems with erectile dysfunction. You agree to switch to an alternative antidepressant. Which of the following would be the most appropriate medication to minimise this adverse effect?

A. Duloxetine
B. Paroxetine
C. Phenelzine
D. Trazodone
E. Venlafaxine

374. A 24-year-old woman with a history of depressive disorder has developed a post-natal depressive episode. She is keen to breastfeed and asks your opinion on an appropriate medication. Which would be your treatment of choice?

A. Doxepin
B. Escitalopram
C. Fluoxetine
D. Nefazodone
E. Paroxetine

371. Answer: D. The most likely diagnosis given the history and exclusion of diabetes mellitus is water intoxication, secondary to illness-related polydipsic behaviour. This has been measured at prevalence rates of 5% in some groups of chronic patients. The diagnosis is based on a history of polydipsia and hyponatraemia at <120 mmol/L. (15, p 582)

372. Answer: B. The patient displays evidence of tardive dyskinesia, more common with typical antipsychotic treatment. The most appropriate treatment would be to switch to an alternative antipsychotic medication. While all of the above have demonstrated some effect, the evidence most strongly supports the use of clozapine. (2, p 99)

373. Answer: D. Most antidepressants have been shown to have a risk of adverse effects on sexual function, be it erectile problems or libido, independent of the underlying depressive illness. With respect to erectile problems alone, all of the above hold varying risk of such, except for trazodone, which can actually be used to promote erections and which also carries a risk of priapism. (2, pp 231–2)

374. Answer: E. All of these antidepressants are excreted in breast milk, and there are reports of mild-to-moderate effects on the infant in some case reports. For newer medications, the evidence base is more limited. Paroxetine is recommended as the antidepressant of choice where pharmacological treatment is indicated. (2, pp 377–80)

375. A 25-year-old woman you have been treating for depression for eight months appears resistant to all trials of pharmacological and psychotherapeutic treatment so far. You have never been able to develop more than a superficial rapport. Her initial attitude of having great faith in your abilities to treat her has now changed to challenging this, not believing you can help her and blaming you for a lack of improvement. She has also indulged in binges of substance abuse, which she later regrets and seeks help for. She has few social supports, having alienated friends with confrontational and erratic behaviour, although she has not been violent towards others. What would be the most likely personality disorder in keeping with the above description?

A. Dissocial personality disorder
B. Dependant personality disorder
C. Emotionally unstable personality disorder
D. Histrionic personality disorder
E. Paranoid personality disorder

376. A 35-year-old man on lithium for one year for the treatment of bipolar disorder is brought to Accident and Emergency by his family due to concerns related to a deterioration in his mental state. Following examination you suspect lithium toxicity. Which of the following would be of most concern?

A. Diarrhoea
B. Coarse tremor
C. Impaired concentration
D. Marked apathy
E. Polydipsia

377. A 45-year-old man with diagnosed alcohol dependence syndrome has had recurrent admissions for detoxification. He has a history of poor self-control due to strong cravings and relapses quickly. He agrees to pharmacological treatment. Which of the following would be the most appropriate?

A. Acamprosate
B. Disulfiram
C. Low-dose chlordiazepoxide
D. Naltrexone
E. Topiramate

378. A 30-year-old woman presents with a six-month history of low mood, associated with low self-esteem, social withdrawal and frequent guilt feelings about her current functional state. Her premorbid function was good, she is in a stable and supportive marriage, there are no relevant major events in her history, and there is no evidence of personality disorder. What form of psychotherapy would be most appropriate for her?

A. Brief psychodynamic psychotherapy
B. Cognitive behavioural therapy
C. Couples therapy
D. Interpersonal psychotherapy
E. Supportive psychotherapy

375. Answer: C.

The constellation of behaviours and schemata, with splitting, impulsivity and poor self-control, episodes of regret and help-seeking, is most in keeping with an emotionally unstable personality. Antisocial personalities are less likely to recognise a problem and regret inappropriate behaviours. Dependant personalities are unlikely to display confrontational behaviours and risk alienating others, wanting to maintain supports as much as possible. Histrionic personalities tend not to risk alienating others, but are instead motivated by desire for positive attention and praise. They are also less regretful, but mainly due to a lack of insight and poor introspection rather than rejection of social norms. The features described in the history are not in keeping with criteria for paranoid personality disorder. (14, pp 934–5)

376. Answer: D.

All of these symptoms are associated with various degrees of toxicity, but marked apathy is the one most associated with severe toxicity. (15, p 36)

377. Answer: A.

Given the instability of his substance use, disulfiram would present too much of a risk to use, or is likely to be discontinued in favour of alcohol use. Acamprosate is the most appropriate and safest licensed medication to use to control cravings. Naltrexone and topiramate have both shown evidence for helping to reduce cravings. Benzodiazepines are not recommended for long-term use. (2, p 315)

378. Answer: B.

Her symptomatology and ideation appear only related to the current depressive episode, and there is no evidence of significant interpersonal difficulties or premorbid traumatic events impacting on her mental state. Supportive therapy may help, but given the strong association between her current cognitive state and her mood, CBT would be the most appropriate model in this case. (14, p 1394)

379. Which of the following agents is most likely to increase clozapine metabolism via induction of CYP1A2?

A. Carbamazepine
B. Cigarette smoking
C. Ciprofloxacin
D. Fluvoxamine
E. Phenytoin

380. A patient has a history of QTc prolongation on sertindole. What would be the most appropriate antipsychotic medication to reduce risk of recurrence of this?

A. Aripiprazole
B. Clozapine
C. Haloperidol
D. Olanzapine
E. Quetiapine

381. An 80-year-old woman with a history of chronic obstructive pulmonary disease and right heart failure, the latter treated with diuretics, presents with depressive disorder. There is no history of stroke. You intend to prescribe a selective serotonin reuptake inhibitor. Which adverse event would you be most concerned about monitoring?

A. Bleeding disorder
B. Diabetes mellitus
C. Hyponatraemia
D. Sedation
E. Urinary retention

382. A patient has not responded to an adequate trial of his current antidepressant treatment. You have recently learned that he was previously treated successfully with tranylcypromine and wishes to use this again. He complied well with necessary requirements of using this previously and you agree to this switch. Based on his current medication, which of the following would be the most appropriate switching regime?

A. On duloxetine – withdraw, wait three weeks, introduce tranylcypromine.
B. On fluoxetine – withdraw, wait three weeks, introduce tranylcypromine slowly.
C. On mirtazapine – withdraw, wait three weeks, introduce tranylcypromine.
D. On moclobemide – withdraw, wait one week, introduce tranylcypromine.
E. On paroxetine – withdraw, wait two weeks, introduce tranylcypromine.

383. A patient with a diagnosis of Pick's disease presents to Accident and Emergency, referred by his general practitioner with suspected Klüver–Bucy syndrome. Which feature is most consistent with this?

A. Childish behaviour
B. Elated mood
C. Hypermetamorphosis
D. Partial seizures
E. Visual hallucinations

379. Answer: B. While having a similar outcome, carbamazepine and phenytoin are CYP3A4 inducers. Ciprofloxacin and fluvoxamine are CYP1A2 inhibitors, leading to reduced metabolism. Cigarettes are recognised to have inducing effects on CYP1A2. (15, p 254)

380. Answer: A. All of the options except for aripiprazole have been seen to confer various degrees of risk, from haloperidol with the highest, then quetiapine, olanzapine and clozapine. (2, p 117)

381. Answer: C. Given her age and her diuretic treatment, there is a high risk of hyponatraemia. While there is some degree of risk of coagulation problems or urinary retention, these would be less likely in this patient. Some degree of reduced risk of diabetes is seen with SSRIs. (2, pp 210–23)

382. Answer: E. It is recommended to wait 1–2 weeks following cessation of most SSRIs, including paroxetine, to ensure adequate washout prior to commencing an MAOI. However, fluoxetine, with an active metabolite norfluoxetine with a half-life of 7-9 days, requires five weeks for adequate washout. Duloxetine only requires one week due its short half-life (12 hours), as does mirtazapine. Tranylcypromine can be commenced 24 hours following cessation of moclobemide, a reversible MAOI. (2, pp 236–9)

383. Answer: C. Hypermetamorphosis (impulsive behaviour of touching things that come into sight) is characteristic of Klüver–Bucy syndrome. The individual would be generally very placid and docile rather than elated. Visual agnosia can occur (inability to recognise objects or faces) but visual hallucinations would not be a feature. Childish behaviour may be a component of Pick's disease, with dysregulation of social conduct and insight into behaviour, but would not be associated with Klüver–Bucy syndrome. (15, p 493)

384. A patient presents to you referred by their general practitioner with depression. You discover that they have been prescribed diazepam for the past four months. Which of the following features would make you most suspicious of dependence?

    A. Evidence of 'doctor shopping' to seek multiple prescriptions.
    B. Gradually increasing dose with no apparent increased tranquilisation.
    C. Regular and frequent use.
    D. Several episodes of cessation but with short-lived success.
    E. Using other benzodiazepines if cannot get diazepam.

385. A patient informs you that the group psychotherapy he is attending for emotionally unstable personality disorder is going well, although he had initially had problems when starting several weeks ago. Which of the following best represents an early stage in the group development?

    A. Deconstruction
    B. Differentiation
    C. Imitation
    D. Independence
    E. Individualisation

386. In Huntington's disease, which of the following is most true?

    A. There is prevalence of 4–9 per 1000 in the UK.
    B. It is an autosomal recessive condition.
    C. Most cases present between the ages of 25 and 35 years.
    D. Two-thirds of initial presentations are for mental rather than physical disorder.
    E. Lifetime suicide risk is approximately 8%.

387. You are asked to see a confused elderly patient on the general medical ward who came in last night. In your assessment, what feature would make you more likely to diagnose a delirium rather than a dementia?

    A. Disorientation
    B. Fluctuating confusion during admission
    C. Hallucinatory phenomena
    D. Impoverished thinking
    E. The patient is alert

388. Which of the following characteristics would most likely suggest an individual would engage well with a cognitive behavioural model of therapy?

    A. Able to clearly describe post-traumatic events.
    B. Able to reflect on thoughts and actions objectively.
    C. Acceptance of transference issues and willingness to explore.
    D. Insightful and accepting of the diagnosis of depression.
    E. Willingness to establish a deep therapeutic relationship.

384. Answer: B.

While all of these items would be consistent with dependence, increased tolerance is the only feature that is diagnostic, in association with other features. It is not clear from the description what the motivation for reinstatement is. This may reflect abuse rather than dependence. (1, pp 75–6)

385. Answer: C.

Options B and C are recognised stages of development in the group process, with imitation forming the earliest stage as individuals start to coalesce and recognise shared features, and differentiation during the final phase as individuals begin to separate from the group identity. Deconstruction may occur later during the internalising phase, as thoughts are reflected on, then reconstructed. (14, p 1453)

386. Answer: E.

Huntington's disease is an autosomal dominant condition, generally presenting between the ages of 35 and 50, which is present in 4–9 per 10 000 of the UK population. Approximately one-third present with mental disorder and two-thirds with physical disorder. Apraxia and agnosia are absent in Huntington's disease. (15, p 517)

387. Answer: B.

All of these features can be present in either condition; however, given the fluctuation in confusion within such a short space of time, this presentation is more consistent with delirium than a dementia. (15, p 512)

388. Answer: B.

Options A, C and E are not necessary features to have for engagement in cognitive behavioural therapy, as it is mainly focused on the 'here and now' symptomatology and rarely requires exploration into deeper and past issues as in psychodynamic therapies. While acceptance of a formal diagnosis of depression is preferred, and is often implied with good engagement, some patients may have a different understanding of the cause for their symptoms. They may still accept and use the CBT model as a means to recovery. (15, pp 129–34)

389. Which of the following is most true with respect to epidemiological measures?

A. Incidence refers to the number of cases present in a population at or within a specific point or period in time.
B. Reliability of a test is the degree to which it measures what it purports to measure.
C. The higher the sensitivity of a test, the lower the false-negative rate.
D. Numerator error is an error in measuring the baseline population from which the cases are taken.
E. Validity is potentially affected if more than one rater administers a test.

390. A prospective mother is concerned about the risk of teratogenicity if she gets pregnant while on lithium. Which of the following best describes the risk of Ebstein's anomaly associated with lithium treatment in pregnancy?

A. 1:10
B. 1:100
C. 1:1000
D. 1:2000
E. 1:500

391. Which of the following is most true about fragile X syndrome?

A. The second most common cause of learning disability
B. X-linked recessive transmission
C. 1:1000 in males and 1:500 in females
D. The second most common inherited cause of learning disability
E. Typical features include small ears and testes

392. A 45-year-old man in the medical ward on linezolid antibiotics developed confusion, muscle rigidity and hyperthermia shortly after he was placed on citalopram for low mood. What is the most likely diagnosis?

A. Serotonin syndrome
B. Drug overdose
C. Alcohol withdrawal state
D. Metabolic disturbance
E. Infective process

393. A 25-year-old female factory worker was treated with risperidone following a three-week history of third-person auditory hallucinations and persecutory delusions. Several days later, she became febrile with fluctuating blood pressure, impaired consciousness and muscle rigidity. What is the most likely diagnosis?

A. Alcohol withdrawal state
B. Neuroleptic malignant syndrome
C. Cholinergic excess
D. Metabolic disturbance
E. Catecholamine excess

389. Answer: C. Option A refers to prevalence, not incidence, which is the number of new cases developing within a specified period. B defines validity, not reliability, which measures the consistency of results obtained on repeating a test (e.g., either at different times or by different raters), thus in option E it is reliability that may be affected. Option D defines denominator error, as the numerator refers to the number of cases, not the total population being examined. (15, pp 698–700)

390. Answer: C. Ebstein's anomaly comprises of dislodgement of the tricuspid valve into the right ventricle. The risk is increased with the use of lithium in the first trimester of pregnancy. Foetal ultrasound and echocardiography are indicated at 16–18 weeks. The risk is 1:1000. (17, p 876)

391. Answer: D. Fragile X syndrome is the second most common cause of learning disability after Down's syndrome, and it is the most common inherited cause of learning disability. Features include learning disability, macro-orchidism, large ears, hypertelorism and blue eyes. (26, p 256)

392. Answer: A. Serotonin syndrome is a rare but serious condition characterised by excess serotonergic activity. Symptoms include confusion, muscle rigidity, hyperreflexia and GI upset. Other symptoms include hyperthermia and fluctuation of blood pressure. Linezolid is an antibiotic used in treatment of gram-positive bacteria. It has weak monoamine oxidase inhibitor, and interaction with selective serotonin reuptake inhibitor has been documented. (27, 29)

393. Answer: B. Neuroleptic malignant syndrome is an idiosyncratic reaction resulting from dopamine antagonism by typical and some atypical antipsychotic medications. It is a rare condition, 0.5% of patients on typical antipsychotic medications have been reported to develop neuroleptic malignant syndrome. It can be life-threatening with a reported mortality rate of 20%. Symptoms include fever, fluctuating blood pressure and fluctuating consciousness. (2, pp 11, 103–6)

394. Which of the following laboratory investigations will help most in arriving at the diagnosis in a patient with suspected neuroleptic malignant syndrome?

    A. Raised creatinine kinase and leucocytosis
    B. Reduced creatinine kinase and leucopenia
    C. Abnormal thyroid function tests
    D. Urinary catecholamine
    E. Serum calcium

395. A 30-year-old petrol attendant with a three-year history of schizophrenia recalled seeing a white cat smiling at him on date 06/06/06, which led to his psychotic symptoms. He strongly believes that date is synonymous with the devil. How is this psychopathology is best described?

    A. A persecutory delusion
    B. A delusional belief
    C. A delusional memory
    D. A delusional mood
    E. A normal belief

396. A 63-year-old man presents with bradykinesia, limb rigidity, unsteady gait, visual hallucinations and fluctuating cognitive impairment on clinical examination. What is the most likely diagnosis?

    A. Lewy body dementia
    B. Alzheimer's dementia
    C. Pick's dementia
    D. Normal pressure hydrocephalus
    E. Delirium

397. Which of the following finding would you most likely expect in a 23-year-old woman who has been diagnosed with anorexia nervosa?

    A. Increased leptin
    B. Decreased cortisol
    C. Increased T3
    D. Increased growth hormone
    E. Increased libido

398. In patients with post-traumatic stress disorder, which of the following statements is most true?

    A. Hyperactivity of medial prefrontal or anterior cingulate networks in regulating the amygdala have been implicated.
    B. Saccadic eye movement control is a useful treatment.
    C. Eye movement desensitisation and reprocessing is a proven treatment (EMDR).
    D. Borderline personality disorder is not a risk factor.
    E. Being male is a risk factor.

394. **Answer: A.**   Serum creatinine kinase is always raised, leucocytosis with a left shift and disordered liver function tests are present. (2, pp 11, 103–6)

395. **Answer: D.**   Delusional memory occurs when a delusion interpretation is given to a normal memory. (29, pp 126–7)

396. **Answer: A.**   Lewy body dementia is characterised by bradykinesia, limb rigidity, unsteady gait, visual hallucination and fluctuating cognitive impairment. (30)

397. **Answer: D.**   Increased growth hormone and cortisol, reduced T3 and libido are common findings in patients with anorexia nervosa. Decreased leptin is associated with anorexia nervosa. (26, p 90)

398. **Answer: C.**   Evidence-based studies have shown the efficacy of eye movement desensitisation and reprocessing (EMDR). Borderline personality disorder and being female are associated risk factors. Underactivity of medial prefrontal or anterior cingulate networks in regulating the amygdala has been implicated. (31)

399. In patients with Parkinson's disease, which of the following is most true?

A. Hypermetabolism in caudate, inferior orbitofrontal and medial frontal regions are observed in positron emission tomography.
B. Dopamine agonists have been implicated in pathological gambling.
C. Auditory hallucinations are major psychotic symptoms.
D. The frequency of psychiatric symptoms is 20%.
E. Hypomania is a major neuropsychiatric disorder.

400. A 40-year-old man with a history of alcohol liver disease presents in an alcohol withdrawal state. Which of the following is your preferred choice of benzodiazepine treatment for his withdrawal symptoms?

A. Diazepam
B. Oxazepam
C. Chlordiazepoxide
D. Flurazepam
E. All of the above

399. Answer: B. There is evidence to suggest that high-dose dopamine agonists are implicated in pathological gambling in patients with Parkinson's disease. Visual hallucinations, persecutory delusions and pathological jealousy are common psychotic symptoms. The frequency of psychiatric symptoms is 70% in patients with Parkinson's disease. (32)

400. Answer: B. Oxazepam is a short-acting benzodiazepine and may be the preferred choice in liver disease in view of the fact that the other types listed are long-acting benzodiazepines and would accumulate in the system, leading to oversedation. Flurazepam is not generally used for alcohol detoxification. (2, p 315)

References

1. World Health Organization. *The ICD-10 Classification of Mental and Behavioural Disorders: clinical descriptions and diagnostic guidelines*. Geneva: World Health Organization; 1992.
2. Taylor D, Paton C, Kerwin R. *The South London and Maudsley NHS Foundation Trust Oxleas NHS Foundation Trust: prescribing guidelines*. 9th ed. London: Informa Healthcare; 2007.
3. Sadock B, Kaplan H, Sadock V. *Kaplan & Sadock's Synopsis of Psychiatry: behavioral sciences*. 10 ed. Philadelphia, PA: Wolter Kluwer/Lippincott Williams & Wilkins; 2007.
4. Johnstone E, Owens D, Lawrie S, Sharpe M, Freeman C. *Companion to Psychiatric Studies*. 7th ed. Edinburgh; New York: Churchill Livingstone; 2008.
5. Stahl S. *Stahl's Essential Psychopharmacology*. 3rd ed. Cambridge: Cambridge University Press; 2008.
6. Sadock BJ, Sadock VA, Kaplan HI. *Kaplan & Sadock's Comprehensive Textbook of Psychiatry*. 8th ed. Philadelphia, PA: Lippincott Williams & Wilkins; 2005.
7. Andreasen N, Black D. *Introductory Textbook of Psychiatry*. Washington, DC: American Psychiatric Publishing; 2006.
8. Puri BK, Hall AD. *Revision Notes in Psychiatry*. London: Arnold; 2004.
9. Wright P, Stern J, Phelan M. *Core Psychiatry*. London: WB Saunders; 2000.
10. Wright P, Stern J, Phelan M. *Core Psychiatry*. 2nd ed. Philadelphia, PA: Elsevier; 2005.
11. Korneva EA, Shanin SN, Rybakina EG. The role of interleukin-1 in stress-induced changes in immune system function. Neurosci Behav Physiol. 2001; **31**(4):431–7.
12. Freeman CPL, Zealley AK. *Companion to Psychiatric Studies*. 6th ed. Johnstone EC, editor. Edinburgh: Churchill Livingstone; 1998.
13. Stein G, Wilkinson G. *Seminars in General Adult Psychiatry*. London: Royal College of Psychiatrists; 1998.
14. Gelder MG, López Ibor JJ, Andreasen NC. *New Oxford Textbook of Psychiatry*. Oxford: Oxford University Press; 2000.
15. Stein G, Wilkinson G. *Seminars in General Adult Psychiatry*: London: RCPsych Publications; 2007.
16. Eysenck M. *Simply Psychology*. Hove, East Sussex, UK: Psychology Press; 1996.
17. Semple D, Smyth R, Burns J, Darjee R, Mc Intosh A. *Oxford Handbook of Psychiatry*. 1st ed. Oxford University Press; 2005.
18. Kaplan H, Sadock B, Sadock V. *Synopsis of Psychiatry: behavioral sciences*. Philadelphia, PA: Lippincott Williams & Wilkins; 2003.
19. Puri B, Hall A. *Revision Notes in Psychiatry*. London: Arnold; New York: Oxford University Press; 1998.
20. Lawlor B. *Revision Psychiatry*. Dublin: MedMedia; 2001.
21. Buckley P, Bird J, Harrison G. *Examination Notes in Psychiatry: a postgraduate text*. Oxford Butterworth-Heinemann; 1995.
22. Singh T, Williams K. Atypical depression. Psychiatry (Edgmont). 2006; **3**(4):33–9.
23. Dayalu P, Chou KL. Antipsychotic-induced extrapyramidal symptoms and their management. Expert Opin Pharmacother. 2008; **9**(9):1451–62.
24. Sadock B, Sadock V. *Kaplan & Sadock's Comprehensive Textbook of Psychiatry*. 7th ed. Philadelphia, PA: Lippincott Williams & Wilkins; 2000.
25. Maj M, Sartorius N, Okasha A, Zohar J. *Obsessive-Compulsive Disorder*. Chichester, UK; Hoboken, NJ: Wiley; 2002.
26. Buckley P, Prewette D, Byrd J *et al*. *Examination Notes in Psychiatry*. 4th ed. Boca Raton, FL: CRC Press; 2003.
27. Huang V, Gortney J. Risk of serotonin syndrome with concomitant administration of linezolid and serotonin agonists. Pharmacotherapy. 2006; **26**(12):1784–93.
28. Morales-Molina J, Mateu-de Antonio J, Marín-Casino M, Grau S. Linezolid-associated serotonin syndrome: what we can learn from cases reported so far. J Antimicrob Chemother. 2005; **56**(6):1176–8.
29. Sims A. *Symptoms in the Mind: an introduction to descriptive psychopathology*. 3rd ed. London: WB Saunders; 2003.
30. Byrne J. Dementia with Lewy bodies. Adv Psychiatr Treat. 1998; **4**(6):360–3.
31. Shapiro F. Eye movement desensitization and reprocessing (EMDR): evaluation of controlled PTSD research. J. Behav Ther Exp Psychiatry. 1996; **27**(3):209–18.
32. Steeves TD, Miyasaki J, Zurowski M *et al*. Increased striatal dopamine release in parkinsonian patients with pathological gambling: a [11C] raclopride PET study. Brain. 2009; **132**(Pt 5):1376–85.

INDEX

A

Absorption rate, drug, 170–1
Acceptability, social, 170–1
Acute intermittent porphyria, 72–3
Adaptive Behaviour Scales, 13
ADHD. *See* Attention deficit hyperactivity disorder (ADHD)
Adjustment disorder, 19
Affect illusions, 19
Affective disorders, 118–9
Agnosias, 116–7
Agomelatine, 90–1
Agoraphobia, 7, 70–1
Agranulocytosis, 28–9, 132–3
Agraphia, 116–7
Akathisia, 3, 172–3
    second-generation atypical antipsychotics and, 108–9
    treatment of, 88–9
Alcohol dependence syndrome, 4
    conditioning and, 8
    disulfiram for, 138–9, 178–9
    employment and, 46–7
    Korsakoff's syndrome and, 14
    during pregnancy, 154–5
    support services, 42–3
    vitamin deficiencies, 44
    Wernicke's encephalopathy and, 134–5
Alcohol liver disease, 188–9
Alexia without agraphia, 104–5
Alprazolam, 54–5, 57
Alzheimer's disease, 67, 119
    epidemiology of, 96–7
    macroscopic changes in, 156–7
    temporal lobe changes with, 166–7
    treatment, 158–9
Ambittendence, 24
Amfebutamone, 54–5
Amino acids, excitatory, 70–1
Amisulpride, 64–7, 106–7
Amitriptyline, 174–5
Amnesia, 15
Amnesic syndrome, 88–9
Amok, 41
Amplification, 166–7

Analytical studies, 126–7
Angelman's syndrome, 60–1
Angina, unstable, 8–9
Anorexia nervosa
    age of onset, 48–9
    biochemical profile in, 26–7
    versus bulimia nervosa, 10–1
    incidence rates, 86–7
    laboratory findings, 186–7
    prognosis, 30–1
Antibiotics, 184–5
Anticholinergic drugs, 34–5
Anticonvulsants, 132–3
Antidepressants, 4, 38–9. *See also* specific drugs
    active metabolites, 56–7
    anti-adrenergic side effects, 56–7
    diabetes mellitus and, 10–1
    erectile dysfunction with, 174–5
    half-lives, 142–3
    hyponatraemia and, 64–5, 150–1
    non-linear pharmacokinetic properties, 54–5
    post-traumatic stress disorder and, 12
    postural hypotension with, 102–3, 150–1
    QTc interval prolonged with, 108–9
    sedation with, 100–1
    sexual side effects of, 7, 12–3, 108–9
    tricyclic, 128–9, 150–1
    unstable angina and, 8–9
    washout period, 54
    weight gain with, 58–9, 150–1
    weight loss with, 174–5
Antipsychotics. *See also* specific drugs
    metabolism, 110–1
    noncompliance, 134–5, 158–9
    QT interval prolonged with, 114–5, 122–3, 180–1
    sedation with, 110–1
    side effects, 170–1
    smoking and, 130–1
    weight gain with, 162–3
Anxiety, 6–7, 14
Apathy, 178–9

Aphasia
  conduction, 160–1
  sensory, 160–1
  transcortical motor, 160–1
Appetite loss, 162–3
Apraxia, 116–7
Aripiprazole, 66–7
  effect on QTc interval, 114–5
  liver metabolism, 102–3
  receptor binding, 88–9
  sedation with, 110–1
Asperger's syndrome, 48–9
Aspirin, 143
Assessment
  intelligence, 172–3
  population level, 174–5
  self-rated, 174–5
Atomoxetine, 102–3
Attachment, 50–1
  difficulties in autistic spectrum disorder, 160–1
Attention deficit hyperactivity disorder
      (ADHD), 60–1
  genetic factors, 124–5
  motor tics and, 102–3
  susceptibility gene, 92–3
Auditory hallucinations, 45
Autistic spectrum disorder, 160–1
Autochthonous delusion, 36–7
Autonomous attachment, 50–1
Autoscopic hallucinations, 13
Autosomal disorders, 58–61, 130–1
Autosomal dominant inheritance, 130–1, 154–5,
      168–9
Availability error, 96–7
Aversion therapy, 138–9
Avoidance symptoms, 32

B
Baby blues, 19
Backward conditioning, 9
Beck Depression Inventory (BDI), 174–5
Bell's palsy, 17
Benzodiazepines, 90–1
  alcohol liver disease and, 188–9
  detoxification from, 4–5
  elimination half-life, 54–5
  opiate withdrawal treatment with, 118–9
  urinary retention and, 9
  withdrawal, 76–7
Bereavement, 23–4
Bias
  confirmation, 96–7

  questionnaire, 8–9
Biofeedback, 138–9
Bipolar affective disorder, 10
  epidemiology, 142–3
  genetics, 100–1
  hypertension with, 132–3
  pregnancy and, 120–1
  relapses, 132–3
  risk in first degree relative of affected
      proband, 92–3
  risk of suicide with, 27
  susceptibility genes, 100–1
  tardive dyskinesia and, 158–9
  tremors and, 46
  versus unipolar depression, 170–1
Blinking, rapid, 12–3
Borderline personality disorder
  childhood emotional difficulties and, 172–3
  eye movement desensitisation and reprocessing
      with, 186–7
  features of, 5–6
  treatment, 140–1
Brain
  fag, 41
  frontal lobe, 160–1, 166–7
  imaging, 156–7, 168–9
  limbic lobe, 174–5
  parietal lobe, 58–9, 122–3, 156–7
  regions, 156–7, 162–3
  tumor, 66–7
Breastfeeding
  benzodiazepines and, 2–3
  lithium and, 120–1
  postnatal depression and, 174–5
Brief Psychiatric Rating Scale, 13
Broca's dysphasia, 9
Bulimia nervosa, 10–1, 122–3
  epidemiology, 154–5
Buprenorphine, 148–9
Bupropion, 102–3

C
CAGE screening tool, 13
Cannabis, 94–5
Capgras syndrome, 25
Carbamazepine
  agranulocytosis and, 132–3
  cytochrome P4502C and, 100–1
  hypersensitivity reaction to, 11
  plasma concentration, 150–1
  prothrombin time and, 102–3
  urinary retention and, 8–9

Caregiver burden, 120–1
CAT. See Cognitive analytical therapy (CAT)
Catalepsy, 32–3
Cataplexy, 32–3
Catatonia, 118–9
Catatonic schizophrenia, 50–1
Cathexis, 32–3
CATIE trial, 62–3
CBT. See Cognitive behavioural therapy (CBT)
Central nervous system development, 112–3
Cerebrovascular accident, 8
Chlormethaziole, 54–5
Chlorphenamine, 57
Chlorpromazine, 64–5
    systemic lupus erythematosus and, 136–7
Chronic interictal psychosis, 74–5
Chronic obstructive pulmonary disease (COPD),
        180–1
Cigarette smoking, 90–1
Cimetidine, 38
Citalopram, 54–5
    active metabolites, 56–7
    post-myocardial infarction use, 102–3
    washout period, 54–5
Clang association, 33
Classical conditioning, 33
Clinical trials, 78–9
Clomipramine, 9, 82–3
Clopenthixol, 54–5
Clozapine, 66–7
    agranulocytosis and, 28–9, 132–3
    metabolism, 180–1
    neutropenia with, 132–3
    pharmalogical properties, 86–7
    as potent agonist, 66–7
    serum prolactin with, 66–7, 90–1
    smoking and, 130–1
Cluttering, 36–7
Cognitive analytical therapy (CAT), 84–5
Cognitive behavioural therapy (CBT)
    for bulimia nervosa, 122–3
    characteristics for success with, 182–3
    for current depressive episode treatment, 178–9
    in early stages of psychosis, 116–7
    as explicit and structured, 152–3
    homework with, 68–9
    for mild depression, 164–5
Cognitive development stages, 140–1
Cognitive dissonance, 46–7
Completion illusions, 19
Compliance therapy, 138–9
Concrete operational stage, 140–1

Condensation, 152–3
Conditioning, 8–9
Conduction aphasia, 160–1
Confirmation bias, 96–7
Contingency, 76–7
Corticospinal tract, 58–9
Couvade syndrome, 7
Cranial nerves, 58–9
Creutzfeldt-Jakob disease, 72–3, 158–9
Cri-du-chat syndrome, 59
Culture-bound syndromes, 40–1
Cytochrome P4502C, 100–1

D
DAMP (deficits in attention, motor control and
        perception), 122–3
DBT. See Dialectical behaviour therapy (DBT)
De Cleramault's syndrome, 7
Deep dysphasia, 160–1
Defence mechanisms, 23–4, 94–5
Delirium, 182–3
Delusional intuition, 36–7
Delusional memory, 36–7, 186–7
Delusional mood, 36–7
Delusional perception, 21
Delusions
    ketamine and, 164–5
    with systemic lupus erythematosus, 136–7
Dementia
    caregiver burden in, 120–1
    delirium versus, 182–3
    early onset, 66–7
    with Lewy bodies, 66–7, 80–1, 186–7
    versus pseudodementia, 148–9
    vascular, 67
Denial, 94–5
Deoxyribonucleic acid (DNA), 128–9
    mutations, 168–9
Dependent personality disorder, 130–1
Depression, 4, 6
    bipolar (See Bipolar affective disorder)
    brains of patients with severe, 82–3
    cannabis and, 94–5
    cognitive behaviour therapy for mild,
        164–5
    electroconvulsive therapy for, 34–5, 46–7,
        48–9
    epidemiology, 142–3
    escitalopram for, 38–9
    failure to respond to medications for, 38–9
    loss of libido and, 12
    "manic," 20

medications and, 28–9
Mendelian mode of inheritance for, 136–7
postnatal, 174–5
post-traumatic stress disorder and, 10–2
poverty and, 140–1
pregnancy and, 18–9
psychosocial vulnerability factors associated with, 140–1
sleep difficulties with, 16–7
treatment-resistant, 112–3
underlying conditions as causes of, 22
unipolar depressive disorder, 62–3, 170–3
unstable angina and, 8
Desensitisation, 138–9
Detoxification, benzodiazepines, 4–5
Dhat, 41
Diabetes mellitus, 10–1
Diagnosis, errors in, 96–7
Dialectical behaviour therapy (DBT), 138–9
Diazepam, 182–3
  bioavailability, 106–7
  half-life, 54–5
DiGeorge syndrome, 136–7
Disorganisation syndrome, 38–9
Disorganised childhood attachment, 50–1
Displacement, 23–4, 94–5
Dissocial personality disorder, 130–1
Disulfiram, 84–5
  prothrombin time and, 102–3
  risks with, 178–9
Diuretics, thiazide, 132–3, 180–1
Dopamine, 124–5
Dosulepin, 100–1
Down's syndrome, 154–5
Doxepin, 100–1
Dream theory, 152–3
Drug development clinical trials, 78–9
Duloxetine, 102–3
Dysbindin, 100–1
Dyskinetic movements, 13
Dyslexia, 60–1
Dysphasia, deep, 160–1
Dysthymia, 6, 118–9
Dystonic movements, 13
  drug-induced, 56–7

E
Early onset dementia, 66–7
Ebstein's anomaly, 184–5
Echolalia, 17, 33, 36–7
ECT. See Electroconvulsive therapy (ECT)

Edinburgh Postnatal Depression Scale, 174–5
Edward's syndrome, 59
Electrocardiogram (ECG), 108–9
Electroconvulsive therapy (ECT)
  anterograde amnesia after, 46–7
  hormonal changes with, 106–7
  medications causing difficulty with, 48–9
  predictors of positive response with, 34–5
  use in schizophrenia, 112–3
Electroencephalogram (EEG)
  epilepsy monitoring, 70–1
  rhythms, 72–3
  sleep cycle, 44–5
  triphasic waves, 120–1
Encephalopathic syndrome, 130–1
Epidemiology
  Alzheimer's disease, 96–7
  bipolar affective disorder, 142–3
  bulimia nervosa, 154–5
  insomnia, 162–3
  investigation levels, 126–7
  measures, 184–5
  post-traumatic stress disorder, 160–1
  suicide, 114–5
  terminology, 80–1
Epilepsy
  EEG and, 70–1
  psychiatric aspects of, 74–5
  relapses, 132–3
  sizures, 42–3
  temporal lobe, 16–7
Erectile dysfunction, 108–9, 174–5
Erickson's psychosexual development stages, 140–1
Escitalopram, 38–9, 54–5
  washout period, 55
Ethical principles of medical treatment, 48–9
Extracampine hallucinations, 6–7
Extrapyramidal pathway, 58
Eye movement desensitisation and reprocessing (EMDR), 186–7

F
Facial nerve, 59
Facial paralysis, 16–7
Falling, risk of, 56–7
Family therapy, 94–5
Fear of abandonment, 130–1
Fetal alcohol syndrome, 154–5
Fetishistic transvestism, 148–9
Fibromyalgia, 40–1

Fire-setting, 68–9
Fluoxetine, 54–55, 57
  bulimia nervosa and, 122–3
  post-myocardial infarction use, 102–3
  postural hypotension with, 150–1
  prothrombin time and, 102–3
  weight loss with, 174–5
Flupenthixol, 29, 54–5, 64–5
Fluphenazine, 54–5, 75
Flurazepam, 188–9
Fluspirilene, 54–5
Fluvoxamine, 102–3
  postural hypotension with, 150–1
Folstein Mini-Mental State Examination,
    114–5
Formal operational stage, 140–1
Fragile X syndrome
  exophenotypic expression, 108–9
  learning disability with, 162–3,
    184–5
  as x-linked recessive disorder, 72–3
Free-association, 152–3
Friedrich's ataxia, 60–1
Frontal lobe damage, 160–1, 166–7
Fronto-temporal dementia, 67
Frotteurism, 148–9
Functional hallucinations, 19
Fundamental attribution error, 96–7

G
Galactosaemia, 60–1
Gender
  affective disorders and, 118–9
  bipolar disorder and, 142–3
  psychiatric disorders and, 23–4
  social phobia and, 92–3
Gender identity disorder, 4–5
General Health Questionnaire, 13
Genetics, 72–3
  attention deficit hyperactivity disorder (ADHD),
    124–5
  bipolar disorder, 100–1
  Down's syndrome and, 154–5
  Huntington's disease, 162–3, 168–9,
    182–3
  puerperal psychosis, 124–5
  relative risk and, 154–5
  schizophrenia, 80–1, 100–1, 116–7, 134–5
  unipolar depressive disorder, 136–7
Gerstmann's syndrome, 26–7, 59, 67,
    168–9
Glasgow Coma Scale, 14–5

Glucocorticoid axis diseases, 22
G-protein receptors, 128–9
Grief reaction, 23–4
Group therapy, 166–7, 182–3

H
Haemodialysis, 56–7
Half-life, drug, 54–5, 142–3
Hallucinations
  auditory, 45
  ketamine and, 164–5
  with schizophrenia, 12–3
  systemic lupus erythematosus and, 136–7
  temporal lobe epilepsy and, 17
  types, 6–7
  visual, 18–9
Haloperidol, 9, 54–5
  cardiac conduction abnormalities with, 122–3
  receptors, 88–9
Haptic hallucinations, 13
Head injury, 114–5
  frontal lobe damage in, 160–1, 166–7
  Rancho Los Amigos Scale (RLAS) and,
    124–5
Heart failure, 180–1
Hemiballismic movements, 13
Heroin dependence, 148–9
Hierarchical Model of Suicide, 156–7
Higher order conditioning, 9
Hunter syndrome, 162–3
Huntington's chorea, 72–3, 114–5
Huntington's disease
  brain imaging, 164–5
  EEG record flattening, 120–1
  genetics, 162–3, 168–9, 182–3
  macroscopic neuropathological changes with,
    166–7
Hygric hallucinations, 13
Hypermetamorphosis, 180–1
Hyperparathyroidism, 11
Hyperreflexia, 65
Hypertension, 132–3
Hypnagogic hallucinations, 6–7, 13
Hypnotic state, 34–5
Hypochondriasis, 35
Hypokalaemia, 100–1
Hyponatraemia
  with antidepressants, 64–5
  with citalopram, 100–1
  risk factors, 150–1
  with SSRIs, 180–1
Hypotension, postural, 102–3, 150–1

I

Immune system and stress, 154–5
Implicit memory, 118–9
Impotence, 6–7
Injury, head, 114–5
Insecure-avoidant attachment, 50–1
Insomnia, 162–3
Intelligence assessment, 172–3
Interpersonal therapy (IPT), 69–70, 138–9
Interviewing, motivational, 74–5
Intoxication, water, 174–5
Intramuscular administration of drugs, 170–1
Intuition, delusional, 36–7
IPT. See Interpersonal therapy (IPT)
IQ tests, 76–7

K

Ketamine, 164–5
Kinaesthetic hallucinations, 13
Klüver–Bucy syndrome, 180–1
Koro, 40–1
Korsakoff's syndrome, 14–5

L

Lamotrigine, 86–7
Latah, 41
Latent content of dreams, 152–3
Learning theory, 76–7
Lesch-Nyhan syndrome, 162–3
Lewy body dementia, 66–7, 80–1, 186–7
Libido, loss of, 12–3, 38–9
    schizophrenia and, 134–5
Likert scale, 8–9
Limbic system, 33, 112–3, 174–5
Linezolid antibiotics, 184–5
Lithium, 9, 54–5, 106–7
    bipolar affective disorder and, 10–1
    breastfeeding and, 120–1
    haemodialysis and, 57
    half-life, 55
    hypertension and, 132–3
    least effective scenarios for, 172–3
    neutropenia and, 132–3
    pregnancy and, 184–5
    toxicity, 178–9
    for treatment-resistant depression, 112–3
    tremors with, 46–7
Liver metabolism, 102–3
Lofepramine, 150–1
Logloclonia, 36–7
Lorazepam, 54–5
    for catatonia, 118–9

M

Malingering
    amnestic disorder and, 44–5
    with schizoaffective disorder, 2
Manic depression, 20
Manifest content of dreams, 152–3
Memory
    delusional, 36–7, 186–7
    implicit, 118–9
    loss, 28, 44
    procedural, 112–3, 148–9
Messenger RNA, 129
Metabolism, drug, 170–1
Metapsychological concepts, 128–9
Methadone, 94–5, 148–9
    safety during pregnancy, 148–9
Methylphenidate, 124–5
Metonymy, 33
Mindfulness-based psychotherapy, 82–3
Minnesota Multiphasic Personality Inventory
        (MMPI), 13, 164–5
Mirroring, 166–7
Mirtazapine, 13, 64–5, 76–7
    sedation with, 100–1
    sexual side effects with, 110–1
Monoamine oxidase inhibitor antidepressants,
        54, 57
Motivational interviewing, 74–5
Movement disorders, 12–3
Multiple sclerosis, 17
Myclonic movements, 13
Myocardial infarction, 102–3

N

Narcissistic personality disorder, 21–2
Narcolepsy, 17
National Comorbidity Survey, 70–1
National Confidential Inquiries into Suicide and
        Homicide by People with Mental Illness,
        142–3
Neurofibromatosis, 60–1
Neurohormones, 126–7
Neuroimaging, 15–7, 168–9
Neuroleptic malignant syndrome (NMS)
    diagnosis, 21–2, 184–5
    mortality rate, 90–1
Neurotransmitters, 70–1
Neutropenia, 132–3
Niemann-Pick disease, 60–1
Nightmares, 32
Night terrors, 17
Noradrenergic receptors, 96–7

O

Obsessive compulsive disorder (OCD), 48–9, 60–1, 68–9
  brain function conditions and, 84–5
  peak incidence of age of onset of, 92–3
  streptococcal infection with, 172–3
  treatment, 120–1
Olanzapine, 64–5, 104–5
  diabetes and, 122–3
  serotonin syndrome with, 22–3
  smoking and, 130–1
Operant conditioning theory, 30–1
Opiate dependence, 94–5
Othello syndrome, 7
Oxazepam, 54–5, 188–9

P

Paliperidone, 158–9
Pallalia, 33, 36–7
Panic disorders, 7, 70–1
Paragrammatism, 36–7
Paralysis, 14–5
  facial, 16–7
  sleep, 32–3
Paranoid personality disorder, 22, 64–5, 178–9
Paranoid schizophrenia, 122–3
  genetics, 116–7
  suicide and, 174–5
  symptoms, 50–1
Pareidolic illusions, 19
Parietal lobe
  lesion, 58–9
  trauma, 122–3
Parkinsonism, medication-induced, 56–7
Parkinson's disease, 88–9
  psychiatric symptoms with, 188–9
Paroxetine, 54–5
  postural hypotension with, 150–1
  sides effects, 128–9
  weight gain with, 58–9
Patau's syndrome, 59
Pathological fire-setting, 68–9
Personality disorders, 20–1, 64–5, 152–3
  borderline, 5, 140–1, 172–3, 186–7
  dependent, 130–1
  DSM classification of, 22
  group psychotherapy for, 182–3
  paranoid, 22, 64–5, 178–9
PET scan, 156–7
Phenelzine, 36–7
Phenylketonuria, 72–3
Phobia, social, 24, 48–9, 92–3

Pick's disease, 114–5, 119, 180–1
Plasma concentration, drug, 158–9
Poliomyelitis, 17
Polymerase chain reaction (PCR), 128–9
Polymorphisms, 128–9
Post-traumatic stress disorder (PTSD), 10–2, 15
  epidemiology, 160–1
  in military veterans, 136–7
  prevalence, 70–1
  psychological therapies to avoid in patients with, 138–9
Postural hypotension, 102–3, 150–1
Poverty and depression, 140–1
Pregnancy
  alcohol use during, 154–5
  bipolar affective disorder and, 120–1
  familial risk of, 22
  lithium use during, 184–5
  methadone use during, 148–9
  puerperal psychosis and, 60–1, 68–9, 134–5
  schizoaffective disorder with, 2–3
Premenstrual syndrome, 60–1
Preoccupied attachment, 50–1
Preoperational stage, 140–1
Primary care settings, 25, 26–7
Procedural memory, 112–3, 148–9
Procyclidine, 106–7
Projection, 94–5
Prolactin, serum, 90–1, 106–7
Prothrombin time, 102–3
Pseudodementia, 28–9, 148–9
Pseudohallucinations, 6–7, 17
Psychiatric Assessment Schedules for Adults with Developmental Disabilities, 174–5
Psychiatric care settings, 26–7
Psychoanalytical theory of mental phenomenon, 128–9
Psychoanalytic thought, 62–3, 152–3
Psychological theory, 62–3
Psychosexual development, Erickson's stages of, 140–1
Psychosis
  chronic interictal, 74–5
  cognitive behavioural therapy (CBT) in in early stages of, 116–7
  puerperal, 60–1, 68–9, 134–5
PTSD. See Post-traumatic stress disorder (PTSD)
Puerperal psychosis, 68–9
  genetics and, 134–5
  onset, 60–1
  prevalence of, 134–5

Q

QTc interval, 108–9
  antipsychotics and, 114–5, 122–3,
    180–1
Questionnaire bias, 8–9
Quetiapine, 64–67, 108–9

R

Ramsay-Hunt syndrome, 17
Rancho Los Amigos Scale (RLAS), 124–5
Rapid eye movement (REM) sleep, 166–7
Reciprocal inhibition, 138–9
Reflex hallucinations, 6–7
Representative error, 96–7
Repression, 94–5
Residual schizophrenia, 50–1
Response prevention, 138–9
Resting membrane ion permeability, 156–7
Restlessness, 2–3
Revision, secondary, 152–3
Rhythms, EEG, 72–3
Ribonucleic acid (RNA), 128–9
Risperidone, 64–7, 184–5
  schizoaffective disorder and, 2–3
  sexual side effects, 134–5

S

Schizoaffective disorder, 2–3
  breastfeeding and, 2
  clang association, 33
  malingering versus factitious disorder, 2
  neutropenia with, 132–3
  urinary retention with, 8
Schizophrenia, 12, 20
  biochemical markers, 174–5
  Capgras syndrome, 25
  catatonic, 50–1
  CATIE trial and treatment of, 62–3
  delusional perception in, 21
  diagnosis, 74–5
  disorganisation syndrome, 38–9
  drug noncompliance, 134–5, 158–9
  familial risk of, 21–2
  genetics and, 80–1, 100–1, 116–7,
    134–5
  involuntary admission for, 48
  medications, 28, 64–5
  movement abnormalities with, 23
  paranoid, 50–1, 116–7, 122–3, 174–5
  post-mortem brains of patients
    with, 78–9
  prevalence, 126–7

  residual, 50–1
  speech disorders, 36–7
  susceptibility genes, 100–1
  thought disorders, 44–5
  treatment-resistant, 132–3
  undifferentiated, 50–1
Schizotypal personality disorder, 22
Seasonal affective disorder, 14–5, 60–1
Secondary revision, 152–3
Secure attachment, 50–1
Sedation
  with antidepressants, 100–1
  with antipsychotics, 110–1
Seizures, 18–9
  epileptic, 42–3
  tricyclic antidepressants and, 128–9
  withdrawal, 5
Selective serotonin reuptake inhibitors (SSRIs), 90–1
  half-lives, 143
  side effects, 128–9
Self-harm, 4, 17, 38. See also Suicide
  dialectical behaviour therapy and, 138–9
  personality assessment and, 164–5
Self-rated assessment tools, 174–5
Sensorimotor stage, 140–1
Sensory aphasia, 160–1
Separation individuation, 172–3
Serotonin
  degradation, 36
  effect on sleep and temperature, 124–5
  receptors, 104–5
  syndrome, 22, 64–5, 184–5
Sertraline, 54–5, 57, 64–5
  weight loss with, 174–5
Serum prolactin, 90–1, 106–7
Sexuality
  disorders, female, 34–5
  drug side effects and, 7, 12–3, 38–9, 108–11,
    174–5
  Erickson's stages of development of, 140–1
  ICD-10 classifications of disorders of, 148–9
  loss of libido, 12–3, 38–9, 134–5
  schizophrenia and, 134–5
Simultaneous conditioning, 9
Sleep
  cycle and EEG, 44–5
  drunkenness, 17
  paralysis, 32–3
  rapid eye movement (REM), 166–7
  serotonin effect on, 124–5
  transitional state between wakefulness and,
    130–1

Smoking, cigarette, 90–1
  schizophrenia and, 130–1
Social acceptability, 170–1
Social phobia, 24, 48–9, 92–3
Sodium valproate, 78–9, 132–3
  as protein bound, 142–3
Somatisation disorder, 30–1, 72–3
Somnambulism, 17
SPECT scan, 156–7
Spinal cord neuroanatomy, 70–1
Spinal trigeminal nucleus, 58–9
Spinothalamic tracts, 70–1
SSRIs. See Selective serotonin reuptake inhibitors
        (SSRIs)
Statistical measures, 126–7
Stimulus conditioning, 9
Streptococcal infection, 172–3
Stress and immune system, 154–5
Subarachnoid haemorrhage (SAH), 94–5
Subcortical auditory dysphasia, 104–5
Sublimation, 94–5
Substance use disorders treatment, 118–9,
        150–1
Suicide, 25, 27, 38–9
  epidemiology, 114–5
  methods, 143
  percentage of people in contact with services
        within week of, 142–3
  predictors of, 156–7, 174–5
  rates, 78–9
Symbolism, 152–3
Systemic lupus erythematosus (SLE), 136–7

T
Tardive dyskinesia
  anticholinergic drugs and, 106–7
  bipolar affective disorder and, 158–9
  prevalence, 32–3
  treatment, 34–5
Temporal lobe
  damage, 80–1
  epilepsy, 16–7
Teratogenicity, 92–3
Thiazide diuretics, 132–3
Thioridazine, 174–5
Tics, 12–13, 16
Tourette's syndrome, 16–7, 48–9, 60–1
Trace conditioning, 9
Transcortical motor aphasia, 160–1
Transcription, RNA, 128–9
Transsexualism, 148–9
Tranylcypromine, 54–5, 180–1

Trauma and classical conditioning, 32–3
Trazodone, 54–5, 90–1, 150–1
Tremors, 46–7
Triazolam, 54–5
Tricyclic antidepressants (TCA), 128–9, 150–1
Tumor, brain, 66–7
Turner syndrome, 59

U
Undifferentiated schizophrenia, 50–1
Unipolar depressive disorder, 62–3
  versus bipolar depression, 170–1
  epidemiology, 142–3
  genetics and, 136–7
  lithium for, 172–3
Unstable angina, 8–9
Upper motor neuron lesion, 15
Urinary retention, 8–9

V
Vaginismus, 35
Vascular dementia, 67
Velocardiofacial syndrome, 136–7
Venlafaxine, 57, 59, 64–5, 108–9
  postural hypotension with, 150–1
Verbigeration, 33
Visual hallucinations, 18–9
Vitamin deficiencies, 44
Voyeurism, 148–9

W
Warfarin, 143
Water intoxication, 174–5
Wechsler Adult Intelligence Scale (WAIS-III),
        172–3
Weight gain
  with antidepressants, 58–9, 150–1
  with antipsychotics, 162–3
Weight loss with antidepressants, 174–5
Wernicke's aphasia, 104–5
Wernicke's dysplasia, 9
Wernicke's encephalopathy, 134–5
Wilson's disease, 60–1, 72–3

Y
Yale-Brown Scale, 174–5

Z
Zaleplon, 90–1
Zolpidem, 90–1
Zopicione, 90–1